# PSYCHOTHERAPY VERSUS BEHAVIOR THERAPY

This volume is published as part of a long-standing cooperative program between Harvard University Press and the Commonwealth Fund, a philanthropic foundation, to encourage the publication of significant and scholarly books in medicine and health.

# PSYCHOTHERAPY VERSUS BEHAVIOR THERAPY

R. Bruce Sloane
Fred R. Staples
Allan H. Cristol
Neil J. Yorkston
Katherine Whipple

A Commonwealth Fund Book
Harvard University Press
Cambridge, Massachusetts
and
London, England

Second printing 1976
Library of Congress Catalog Card Number 75-778
ISBN 0-674-72228-0
Printed in the United States of America

This book is dedicated to
**Mike Serber**
who would have hated it.

ACKNOWLEDGMENTS

This work was carried out with the help of Mental Health Grant Number 15493-01 from the Department of Health, Education and Welfare. A Commonwealth Fund grant-in-aid contributed toward its completion.

We are deeply grateful to Doctors Herbert Freed, Arnold A. Lazarus, Michael Serber, Jay Urban, Raul H. Vispo, and Joseph Wolpe without whose unstinting help this study could not have been completed. Mrs. Olga Aigner and Mrs. Diana Horvitz provided unswerving devotion as research assistants. We thank Mrs. June Payne, who bore the first brunt of the manuscript, and Theo Nicholas, who with the help of Judy Refsland brought it to completion.

Last but not least we thank our patients whose cooperation was so crucial. Their names and personal descriptions have been changed to prevent identification.

## CONTENTS


Foreword by Judd Marmor, M.D. xv
Foreword by Joseph Wolpe, M.D. xix
1. Introduction 1
2. How Psychotherapy Has Been Studied 15
3. The Plan of the Study 49
4. Outcome of Treatment at Four Months 87
5. Follow-Up Evaluations 117
6. Differences Between Behavior Therapy and Psychotherapy 145
7. Patient Characteristics, Process Measures, and Outcome 173
8. Summary 215
Appendices
1 Structured and Scaled Interview to Assess Maladjustment (SSIAM) 229
2 Method of Random Assignment to Groups 235
3 Stipulative Definitions of Psychotherapy and Behavior Therapy 237
4 Two-Tailed and One-Tailed t Tests 241
5 Lennard and Bernstein Scale of Therapist Informational Specificity 243
6 Regression Transformation 245
Notes 247
Index 261

## TABLES

1 MMPI Clinical Scale Scores of Patient Groups at Initial Assessment 61
2 Psychometric Scores of Patient Groups at Initial Assessment 63
3 Number of Target Symptoms in Each Context 65
4 Number of Each Kind of Target Symptom 67
5 Number of Target Symptoms in Each Area of Functioning 68
6 Severity of Target Symptoms: Initial Assessor Ratings 69
7 Number of Patients in Each Treatment Subgroup 76
8 Univariate and Multivariate F Values of Target Symptom Change 89
9 Analyses of Variance of Four-Month Change Scores 94
10 Analyses of Variance of Four-Month Change Scores: Patients in Active Treatment Groups 96
11 Changes in Anxiety at Four Months: Analyses of Variance 99
12 Target Symptom Severity and Overall Adjustment at Four Months: Analyses of Variance of Patient Comparative Ratings 106
13 Work, Social, and Sexual Adjustment at Four Months: Analyses of Variance of Patient Comparative Ratings 106

14 Patients Receiving Treatment Between Four-Month and One-Year Assessments 120
15 Analyses of Variance of One-Year Change Scores for all Patients 124
16 Patients Receiving Further Treatment Compared with Those Who Did Not: Self-Rating of Target Symptoms, Work, and Social Adjustment 126
17 Patients Receiving Further Treatment Compared with Those Who Did Not: Demographic and Personality Characteristics 128
18 Changes from Initial to One-Year Assessment in Patients Receiving No Further Treatment 132
19 Target Symptom Severity and Overall Adjustment at One Year: Analyses of Variance of Comparative Ratings by Patients 138
20 Work, Social, and Sexual Adjustment at One Year: Analyses of Variance of Comparative Ratings by Patients 139
21 Target Symptom Severity and Overall Adjustment at One Year for Patients Who Received No Further Treatment: Analyses of Variance of Comparative Ratings by Patients 140
22 Work, Social, and Sexual Adjustment at One Year for Patients Who Received No Further Treatment: Analyses of Variance of Comparative Ratings by Patients 141
23 Demographic Characteristics and Outcome 189

A-1 Examples of SSIAM Scales 232

## FIGURES


1 Severity of Target Symptoms at Initial and Four-Month Assessment: Rated by Assessors 88
2 SSIAM Work and Social Pathology at Initial and Four-Month Assessment: Rated by Assessors 93
3 Change in Anxiety at Four Months: Rated by Assessors 98
4 Target Symptom Severity at Four Months: Rated by Assessors 102
5 Overall Adjustment at Four Months: Rated by Assessors 102
6 Change in Target Symptoms at Four Months: Rated by Patient 104
7 Overall Improvement at Four Months: Rated by Patient 105
8 Improvement at Four Months by Area: Rated by Patient 107
9 Different Raters' Estimates of Improvement for Behavior Therapy Patients 109
10 Different Raters' Estimates of Improvement for Psychotherapy Patients 110
11 Different Raters' Estimates of Improvement for Wait List Patients 111

12 Target Symptom Severity: Assessor Ratings of all Patients 122
13 Work Inadequacy: Assessor SSIAM Ratings of All Patients 122
14 Social Isolation: Assessor SSIAM Ratings of All Patients 123
15 Target Symptom Severity: Assessor Ratings of Patients Who Received No Treatment after Four Months 130
16 Work Inadequacy: Assessor SSIAM Ratings of Patients Who Received No Treatment after Four Months 130
17 Social Isolation: Assessor SSIAM Ratings of Patients Who Received No Treatment after Four Months 131
18 Improvement at One Year for All Patients: Rated by Patients 137
19 Improvement at One Year for Patients Who Received No Treatment after Four Months: Rated by Patients 138
20 Truax Variables for Behavior Therapists and Psychotherapists During Fifth Interview 148
21 Therapist Informational Specificity Ratings During Fifth Interview 152
22 Therapist and Patient Speech and Pause Times 153
23 Therapist and Patient Speech Units and Interruptions 154
24 Therapist and Patient Speech Durations and Reaction Times 155
25 Frequency of Therapist Statements in Each Content Category During Fifth Interview 159
26 Therapist Attitude Toward the Patient 161
27 Patient Ratings of Therapists on the Relationship Questionnaire 163
28 Patient Rating of Therapist Behavior (Lorr Scale) 164
29 Truax Ratings of Individual Therapists 167

30 MMPI and Treatment Outcome for Psychotherapy Patients 177
31 MMPI and Treatment Outcome for Behavior Therapy Patients 178
32 MMPI and Treatment Outcome for Wait List Patients 179
33 Treatment Outcome for Patients with High Initial MMPI Scores 180
34 Treatment Outcome and Initial Level of Severity 181
35 Treatment Outcome and Severity of Initial Disturbance 182
36 Personality Measures and Treatment Outcome: Psychotherapy Patients 183
37 Personality Measures and Treatment Outcome: Behavior Therapy Patients 184
38 Personality Measures and Treatment Outcome: Wait List Patients 184
39 Outcome for Patients with High Scores on Selected Personality Characteristics 185
40 Kinds of Symptoms and Treatment Outcome 186
41 Contexts of Symptoms and Treatment Outcome 187
42 Modes of Action of Symptoms and Treatment Outcome 188
43 Truax Variables and Treatment Outcome: Psychotherapy Patients 191
44 Truax Variables and Treatment Outcome: Behavior Therapy Patients 191
45 Speech Characteristics and Treatment Outcome: Psychotherapy Patients 193
46 Speech Characteristics and Treatment Outcome: Behavior Therapy Patients 194
47 Therapist Informational Specificity and Treatment Outcome: Psychotherapy Patients 195

48 Therapist Informational Specificity and Treatment Outcome: Behavior Therapy Patients 196
49 Temple Content Categories and Treatment Outcome: Psychotherapy Patients 197
50 Temple Content Categories and Treatment Outcome: Behavior Therapy Patients 199
51 Psychotherapist Attitude Toward Patients and Treatment Outcome 200
52 Behavior Therapist Attitude Toward Patients and Treatment Outcome 201
53 Relationship Questionnaire and Treatment Outcome: Psychotherapy Patients 202
54 Relationship Questionnaire and Treatment Outcome: Behavior Therapy Patients 203
55 Patient Perception of Psychotherapist Behavior (Lorr Scale) and Treatment Outcome: Psychotherapy Patients 204
56 Patient Perception of Behavior Therapist Behavior (Lorr Scale) and Treatment Outcome: Behavior Therapy Patients 205

# Foreword

by
Judd Marmor, M.D.

The evaluation of the results of psychotherapy is one of the most challenging problems facing contemporary behavioral science researchers. What constitutes psychotherapeutic change, let alone what causes it, continue to be issues of considerable ambiguity. The magnitude of the research task becomes compounded geometrically when, in addition, efforts are made to compare the efficacy of differing therapeutic techniques with one another. The question of whether matched samples of emotionally disturbed persons are truly achievable, the issue of adequate controls, the extent to which random and fortuitous life events influence the therapeutic outcomes, and a host of other variables, all present problems of enormous complexity. Add to these the difficulties of assessing and comparing the work not only of different psychotherapists but also of the assessors themselves, and one begins to appreciate the reasons for the paucity of sound research in this area.

The authors of the present study, however, have firmly grasped the prickly nettles involved in these troublesome issues and have handled them with rare lucidity and judicious objectivity. The results of their research are both sobering and reassuring to behavior therapists as well as to psychoanalytically oriented psychotherapists, and offer little comfort to those adherents of either group who are involved in passionately proclaiming the inherent superiority of their particular brand of therapy over all others. The authors' findings suggest that both types of therapy work about equally well, each with only slight advantage for certain types of problems. There is, moreover, considerable overlap, by the therapists' own admission, in the techniques of both groups. Among other things, both groups take detailed psychiatric histories, both attempt to formulate the patients' problems and to reconstruct possible original causes for them, both look for continuing causes in the present, both correct misconceptions, elucidate objectives, and make use of abreaction and of suggestion. Many of the differences are matters of degree rather than of substance. Behavior therapists tend in general to be more directive, more active, more concerned with symptoms and less concerned with childhood memories than are the dynamic psychotherapists. Interestingly, the behavior therapists made virtually the same number of interpretive statements as did the psychotherapists. This is not to say there are not also notable technical differences between them, such as the deliberate behavioral-training techniques of the behavior therapists, or the focused concern of the psychoanalytic therapists with transference reactions and dream interpretations.

Nevertheless, the question of whether the two groups of therapists in this study used two basically different approaches to reach the same therapeutic end, or whether the effectiveness of their treatments was in fact due to factors common to both approaches rather than to their specific theoretical orientations, remains unresolved. There is much in the present study to suggest that the latter may indeed have been the case. Thus the successful patients in *both* groups placed the emphasis for their improvement on the same factors: (1) The personality of the therapist (*relationship*)—patients in both groups who perceived a greater nonpossessive warmth and awareness in their therapists tended to improve more. (2) His helping them to understand their problems (*insight*). (3) His encouraging them to practice facing things that had been bothering them (*practice - "working through"*). (4) Being able to talk to an understanding person (*catharsis, trust*). (5) Helping them to greater self-understanding (*insight*).

These patient-perceptions correspond roughly to the factors that I have set forth in some of my own publications as the primary factors common to all psychotherapies. They are: (1) *Release of tension,* through catharsis and by virtue of the patient's hope, trust, and expectancy. (2) *Cognitive learning* (insight), both by trial and error and by gestalt. (3) *Operant conditioning*, by virtue of manifest (in behavior therapies) or covert (in dynamic psychotherapies) reward-punishment cues from the therapist, as well as by "corrective emotional experiences" (Franz Alexander) in the psychotherapeutic relationship. (4) *Identification with the therapist* (A good example of this in the present study is the statement by one of the patients, Tom, that "he liked his therapist's philosophy of life very much and this helped to crystallize his own." In this instance the patient had some awareness of the identification that had taken place but more often the process is an unconscious one. The fact, moreover, that Tom's therapist was a behavior therapist underlines the point that such identification takes place in behavior therapy no less than in dynamic psychotherapy.) (5) *Reality testing*, which dynamic psychotherapists call "working through," and which is the equivalent of practice in the learning process.

Like any good research, the present study raises as many questions as it answers. One, suggested by the authors themselves, is whether the slightly better results (albeit statistically insignificant) achieved by the behavior therapists are a reflection of the fact that behavioral techniques may be better suited to the arbitrary four-month time limitation imposed on the therapies in this study—that, among other things, patients treated behaviorally were more likely to feel they had had a fair trial and to feel less frustrated when their treatment was cut off. Another is the question of whether the degree of activity of the therapist in and of itself may not be a significant therapeutic variable. Therapist activity may have many unconscious meanings for the patient, most important of which may be the fact that it represents a kind of symbolic giving on the part of the therapist as well as an affirmation of his ongoing interest, concern, and effort to be helpful.

This is a study that will be referred to again and again in all future psychotherapeutic research. It is a model for further efforts in this direction, and in its perceptive conclusion "that the temple of truth may be approached by different pathways" it offers renewed hope to all who are struggling laboriously to gain a glimpse of that glittering edifice.

# Foreword

by
Joseph Wolpe, M.D.

Although I participated in some early planning meetings for the study that this book describes, and although I was involved as "a behavior therapist" in the study, I did not realize what a splendid piece of research had been in the making until I saw the final manuscript. In the perceptiveness of its planning, the variety and rigor of its comparisons, and the care of its execution, it is unmatched by any other clinical study in the history of psychotherapy. The experiment is described in this book in a style so smooth and compelling that I read the manuscript from beginning to end, practically without pause.

The comparison between behavior therapy and brief psychoanalytically-oriented psychotherapy that was the central purpose of the study was statistically inconclusive, but a wealth of information was obtained that will be indispensable to researchers in psychotherapy for years to come. Some interesting trends were found. There were indications that in the more severely disturbed patients behavior therapy was more effective, though in milder cases both approaches were in equal measure superior to a "no treatment" control. There may be a parallel to this in the finding, in recent studies on small animal phobias, that almost any program of psychotherapeutic intervention is effective in overcoming mild neuroses, in contrast to the fact that explicit conditioning techniques are significantly superior in the treatment of major neuroses. I predict that future research will show that the more severe the neurosis, the more significant will be the superiority of behavior therapy over psychoanalytically-oriented psychotherapy or any other system of therapy that does not make explicit use of experimentally established principles relevant to behavior change.

Apart from these intimations of future findings, this book is also sure to benefit the public image of behavior therapy by its dispassionate testimony to the fact that behavior therapists are no less human and humane than therapists of other orientations. The fact that the methods of behavior therapy are based on lawful relations that have largely emerged from animal studies often elicits the illogical inference that behavior therapists treat their patients coldly and restrictively and without interest in the breadth and depth of human experience. This belief is strongly contradicted by some of the findings of this study. In point of fact, the great advances of modern medicine have almost all been based on knowledge of lawful relations in the human organism, and there is no reason to believe that increasing the power of the therapist to produce beneficial change decreases his humaneness.

Although the foregoing remarks have concentrated on behavior therapy, the results of the study were by no means one-sided, and there is much in the book that will give gratification and comfort to the psychoanalysts as well.

# PSYCHOTHERAPY VERSUS BEHAVIOR THERAPY

# 1 Introduction

Psychotherapy is a slippery subject to study. Merely to ask such a seemingly straightforward question as "Is psychotherapy effective?" requires a series of definitions and explanations of points that would be obvious to anyone studying an analogous question like "Does drug therapy work?" It is not easy to answer the questions "What do you mean by psychotherapy?" "Effective with what kind of patients?" "What do you mean by effective?" And the definitions chosen may strongly influence the results.

The research reported here was designed, first, to provide evidence about whether short-term psychotherapy "works" with outpatients and, if so, whether analytically oriented therapy or behavior therapy works better; second, to gather information about the similarities and differences between the two therapies; and third, to identify other factors influencing therapeutic outcome. We will first discuss some of the assumptions and definitions upon which this research rests. The reader will find later, in Chapter 2, a survey of the relevant literature, intended to provide the necessary background for the problem and to clarify our reasons for studying certain aspects of it.

## PATIENTS

People who come to psychotherapists are nearly always unhappy, and they come seeking relief for their unhappiness. If the patient is so seriously disturbed that he cannot care for himself or is physically dangerous to himself or others, he is likely to be called schizophrenic or psychotic, to become an inpatient, and to have drugs or shock treatments as an important part of his therapy. If he is not dangerous and can take care of himself, he is more likely to be called a neurotic or a personality disorder and to be treated as an outpatient, largely with a "talking therapy."

This distinction between patients who should be hospitalized and others who can better be treated as outpatients is an important and useful one, and experienced psychotherapists can generally agree on which group a given patient falls in. But psychiatric diagnosis is still a crude art, and at finer levels of distinction the differences in definition, etiology, treatment of choice, and prognosis between different disorders become so vague as to be practically meaningless. Geertsma and Stoller, for example, found almost no agreement among twenty-seven experienced psychotherapy instructors who filled out long questionnaires describing observationally, diagnostically, prognostically, and psychodynamically two patients whom they had just seen in filmed psychiatric interviews.[1] Their disagreement was not only as to degree of disturbance, but as to the very presence or absence of specific symptoms and behaviors.

There is, for example, such a variety of definitions of the neurotic, the typical outpatient, that it would be difficult indeed for the naive observer to enter the jungle of psychopathology and emerge bearing a neurotic patient. In Kolb's standard textbook description, the psychoneuroses form a connecting link between the various adaptive devices unconsciously utilized by the average mind and the extreme, often disorganized, methods observed in the psychotic.[2] The symptoms of these disorders are either manifestations of anxiety, directly felt and expressed, or efforts to control anxiety. The control defenses include conversion, dissociation, displacement, phobia formation, and repetitive thoughts and acts. In the psychoneuroses, Kolb says, repression is never complete enough to prevent both the feeling and manifestation of anxiety and the formation of unconscious repetitive techniques designed to control it. Other authors emphasize the types of behavior, described by Redlich and Freedman as inappropriate, inadequate, unadaptive, and infantile[3], by which neurotics can be detected, or they stress the cause of the disorder such as conflicts between inner psychological states.

Nearly all descriptions of the neuroses involve anxiety, and anxiety is in fact the chief characteristic of the neuroses in the classification of the American Psychiatric Association.[4] But the personality disorders, the next most common of outpatient problems, although defined in different ways, may have apparently similar etiologies, and often cannot be differentiated reliably from the neuroses by expert diagnosticians. The personality disorders are not thought to cause anxiety, but most patients so diagnosed do report anxiety. Their symptoms are supposed to be gratifying, or "ego-syntonic," as compared with the neurotics' "ego-dystonic" ones, but it seems unlikely that a patient would seek to be rid of a symptom which caused him only pleasure.

For the pharmacologist to test his new drug on the first hundred patients who set foot in his clinic, without inquiring whether or not they had the specific disease his drug was intended to cure, would be ridiculous. Yet this is not far from the best that students of psychotherapy can do. With few exceptions—such as severe phobias, which are easily diagnosed, and whose treatment of choice may prove to be systematic desensitization—we cannot yet diagnose nonpsychotic disorders specifically enough to test hypotheses about treatments of choice for given syndromes. In this study patients were classified along a number of dimensions, including traditional psychiatric diagnoses, in the hope that diagnostic types that were particularly susceptible to one treatment or another would appear. The composition of our sample in terms of these classifications is described in later chapters. In simpler terms, the patients in this study were "typical outpatients."

## EFFECTIVENESS OF TREATMENT

The effectiveness of a treatment measures its success in reaching its goals, and the goals of psychotherapy seem obvious. Apart from the occasional patient with no apparent problem but a desire to enrich his experience and intensify his self-knowledge (and these were excluded from this study), a patient nearly always seeks relief from "problems of an emotional nature."[5] Criteria of improvement, standards of "removal of unhappiness," also seem obvious, except for the serious difficulties in quantifying and reliably measuring such changes. The first possibility is to ask the patient if he is feeling better. This has the advantage of simplicity but the same disadvantage—it may be so simple and vague as to lack meaning. Another way is to measure symptomatic improvement. This has the major advantage of relative objectivity; judgments are confined to circumscribed areas, and the patient himself is permitted to choose in advance which areas those will be. The success of therapy is measured in terms of its effectiveness in changing the things the patient wanted changed when he sought treatment. Such information is useful, and in fact formed the major outcome measure of this study, but taken by itself it is not enough.

The reasons are several. First, a patient may be educated to accept his symptoms rather than be cured of them, and this is not just so much professional hocus-pocus. For example, if a therapist can convince a patient that masturbation, say, or occasional anger at his mother, is perfectly normal, he may entirely cure the problem without altering the symptom in the least. Second, many therapists, especially psychoanalysts, believe that symptomatic improvement does not necessarily signal improvement of the deeper problem underlying the symptom. If symptoms are driven underground without accompanying deep improvement, symptom substitution is likely to occur. The underlying problem then may cause a new, possibly more severe symptom to take the place of the old. However, a successful psychoanalysis is usually accompanied by symptomatic improvement. Strupp has argued against the concept of psychotherapy as a technique for the removal of specific symptoms.[6] In his study, patients who benefited from psychotherapy said their interpersonal functioning was improved and that they had better self-esteem and a greater interest in living, with more energy and satisfaction. They had a greater sense of mastery, felt themselves more able to solve effectively the problems of life, and had a better capacity to make sound judgments based on realistic appraisal of the facts at hand.

It is interesting that they had not complained much of such deficiencies when initially assessed. Improvement in anxiety and depression, of which they had frequently complained, was less frequent. Such increased "adjustment," clearly an important goal of therapy, may occur more or less independently of symptomatic improvement. Unfortunately it is somewhat more difficult to measure than symptomatic improvment. In this study general adjustment was measured by the Structured and Scaled Interview to Assess Maladjustment.[7] This consists of a series of specific questions about several aspects of the patient's adjustment, about his work and his social and sexual life, for example. We used other, less important indices of change, such as the severity of anxiety, but improvement in target symptoms and in overall adjustment were the principal measures. These of course give no direct impression of unconscious or underlying change, but no objective measure could do so.

In later chapters we discuss in more detail the important question of who is to judge therapeutic progress. The therapist may have a natural tendency to find his own treatment successful, and his standards of improvement will inevitably be influenced by his therapeutic beliefs. A behavior therapist might give high marks to a patient whose symptoms had disappeared, whether or not he understood why. A psychotherapist might consider himself successful if his patient thoroughly understood and could better handle his symptoms, even if they remained. Neither view is necessarily right or wrong, but the two cannot properly be compared as the sole measure of effectiveness of their respective treatments. The patient's own evaluation of his improvement is obviously most important, but his report also may be biased in either direction, perhaps because he loves or loathes his therapist. It is difficult to get a large number of patients to report results consistently, so that they can be compared on the same scale; one man's "severe" is another man's "mild."

For these reasons the major data of this study were ratings made as objectively and consistently as possible by three assessors. These psychiatrists tried to remain blind to what treatment the patient had had and gained all their information only from the patient. Supplementary ratings made by the therapist and by the patient himself were compared to the assessor's ratings. Judgments made by a close friend or relative of the patient were also compared. These could provide more independent ratings of the patient as he was "in real life" than could the therapist or the assessor who knew only what the patient told them. Both deliberately and unintentionally, patients have hoodwinked even the most experienced psychiatrist. Moreover, a patient is not an island unto himself. A treatment which makes him feel marvelous may seem disastrous and cause catastrophe to those he lives and works with. We hoped the informants' ratings would make us aware of such effects if they occurred.

## TYPES OF PSYCHOTHERAPY

In 1959 Harper described thirty-six different kinds of psychotherapy.[8] His list was not exhaustive even at that time, and since then many new therapies have emerged, each with a different name, underlying theory, and set of therapeutic strategies. Advocates of each believe its novel approach is far superior to others if not in fact the final answer to the problem. Janov modestly describes his new treatment "Primal Therapy, The Cure for Neurosis."[9] The old Army rule ("If it works, it's obsolete") holds true here; as soon as a new therapy has attracted more than a tiny handful of fanatical supporters, and has reached a point where its effectiveness could be systematically studied, a zealot starts drastically improving upon it. He is usually too busy developing new methods to do any empirical tests. If he does report results, they are repudiated by therapists loyal to the old sect on the ground that he isn't really doing Therapy X any more. After mutual recriminations he will come to agree and declare himself to have founded Therapy Y at which time the whole mitotic process begins again. In an effort to avoid the Humpty-Dumpty aura which often results, in which the word psychotherapy means exactly what the speaker means it to mean, behavior therapy and analytically oriented psychotherapy are briefly described in the next pages.

## PSYCHOANALYTICALLY ORIENTED PSYCHOTHERAPY

The psychotherapeutic method most frequently used in America today is the psychoanalytically oriented approach. Such therapy uses the theoretical framework provided by psychoanalysis. Two major assumptions in the psychoanalytic approach are that unconscious mental processes exist and that the analyst has a role in interpreting them. He points out the components and origins of the patient's conflicts, and their hidden connections, to produce insight and make these conflicts conscious.

Certainly psychoanalysis as a treatment in its classical form is complex and, as Redlich observes, does not lend itself to brief presentation. However, psychoanalytically oriented psychotherapy is somewhat easier to describe. Current personality dynamics are likely to receive the greatest emphasis in this form of therapy. There is less concern with a detailed reconstruction of the patient's past life, and the therapeutic goals are less extensive than in psychoanalysis. However, even the most present-oriented therapist deals to some extent with the past and its effect on the patient.[10]

Redlich cuts through much of the verbiage surrounding the topic by a concise description of what he calls "a common brand of dynamic psychotherapy." Patients are seen in a fifty-minute hour, usually one to three times a week, extending over months or years. The patient usually sits opposite the therapist and talks of his thoughts, feelings, and experiences. Such talk usually leads to the topic of his emotions, anxiety, guilt, or shame, of which he may be unaware.

Redlich stresses the importance of the patient's motivation and the specificity and concreteness of interpretation and clarification. He believes that sensitive accepting, listening, and timely interpretation are the main tools, and that insight achieved in the therapeutic session needs to be applied in real life. He points out that in a permissive relationship the patient may begin to feel, say, and understand what was not consciously felt and understood before. Finally, Redlich emphasizes that the therapist should be aware of his own feelings toward the patient.

## BEHAVIOR THERAPY

Behavior therapy assumes that the patient's maladaptive behavior, which is itself termed the "neurosis," represents efforts to reduce anxiety by escape, avoidance, and other means. Such symptoms, like all other behaviors, are maintained by their effects. Although this approach borrows heavily from the learning theories, there is no single such theory, and therapeutic need often outweighs science. A common brand of behavior therapy has not yet evolved, but three main techniques are desensitization, aversion, and operant conditioning.

### *Desensitization*

Desensitization is a counter-conditioning technique. Relaxing, aggressive, sexual, or other responses that are antagonistic and therefore inhibitory to anxiety are systematically evoked in the presence of the anxiety-producing thoughts or stimuli. This "reciprocal inhibition" gradually weakens the bond between these stimuli and the anxiety.

Important to this approach is the construction of an "anxiety hierarchy," a list of stimuli on a common theme, arranged according to the amount of anxiety they evoke. Working from the patient's history and from information provided by questionnaires, the therapist helps the patient to enumerate these stimuli and the situations which provoke fear. The clinical skill involved in deciding both theme and hierarchy is probably crucial for the success of the treatment.

Assertive training, a variety of desensitization, makes use of self-assertion, which is antagonistic to anxiety and which can easily be invoked in social situations. Those who suffer from interpersonal anxiety evoked by the behavior, attitudes, or opinions of others respond well and rapidly to this procedure. The patient is encouraged to stand up for himself, to express his spontaneous emotions freely, and to voice legitimate differences of opinion rather than to simulate agreement. He is taught to accept and express praise and to improvise and act spontaneously. Assertive acts that might have seriously punishing consequences for the patient are never instigated. It is likely that the expression of positive emotional feeling reciprocally inhibits the anxiety that the patient normally experiences in the anxiety-producing social situation.

Therapeutic sexual arousal is another variety of this technique. Sexual responses, like relaxation, are theoretically incompatible with anxiety and may be used to inhibit anxiety. This technique finds its widest application in the treatment of sexual fears, especially impotence and frigidity. The patient is instructed to terminate any sexual activity as soon as anxiety is detected. He is told to engage in gradual sexual activity when the positive desire is present, and to cease sexuality and induce relaxation if and when anxiety arises. Positive sexual activities are self-reinforcing when anxiety is avoided by these means.

### *Aversion Therapy*

Aversion therapy teaches by punishment. The aversive stimulus is contingent on the occurrence of the deviant behavior.

The most common use of such an approach has been in sexual perversions. When the deviant stimulus evokes sexual arousal, as painful electric shock is administered. Such treatment may be effective because it conditions anxiety to the deviant sexual stimulus and to the internal response stimuli associated with the performance of the deviant behavior.

### *Operant Conditioning*

In this kind of conditioning, behavior is brought under the control of its consequences, namely reward or nonreward. Habits are established by presentation of positive reinforcement or reward following the desired behavior.

First, it is essential to devise a reward system that can produce a high level of response over a considerable period of time. Without an adequate incentive, behavioral control is likely to remain weak and unstable. Money, success, possessions, privilege, and approval, with or without associated affection, are some of the more common human motivations. Self-approval is also an important motivator. Many persons who seek psychiatric treatment are dissatisfied with themselves despite an adequate social repertoire.

Second, it is important that the reinforcing events be made conditional upon the occurrence of the desired behavior. Reinforcement is commonly used to modify behavior in real life, but it may have little effect because its poor timing reinforces the wrong response. Even when appropriate rewards are made at the correct time, they may be only sporadically applied.

Third, methods must be arranged that will produce the desired responses often enough for them to become well established. Behavior can be gradually shaped by selective reinforcement of successively closer approximations to the desired pattern. However, in humans it is likely that such behavior can more quickly be elicited by providing instructions about the desired goal or by having someone act as a model of the desired behavior. There is evidence that autonomic responses as well as overt behavior can be brought under control if reinforced.

Extinction is the progressive weakening of a response when it is not reinforced.

Operant conditioning has been widely used in closed institutions but is less common in "one-to-one" behavior therapy. However, it is likely that the therapist's reinforcement largely shapes what the patient says or does not say in both traditional and behavioral psychotherapy. In this way the approval or nonapproval of the therapist modifies the patient's reports and subtly, or not so subtly, transmits to him the attitudes of the therapist, his mores, and his goals. The welcome sight of a head nodding in agreement with one's own statements serves as a simple, everyday illustration of the effects of reinforcement. Undoubtedly such factors greatly influence psychotherapy. Nevertheless, it is likely that they are used, if not randomly, certainly in a way which may limit their effectiveness. Reinforcements undoubtedly help the therapist to transmit his rationale of therapy to the patient. If the patient agrees with this rationale he is more likely to benefit from treatment than if he rejects it. It has been suggested that an important part of "insight" derives from such sharing of views and their acceptance by the patient. The behaviorist's theoretical framework makes him more likely to use such techniques consciously than a psychotherapist, who is likely to eschew "control."

Psychoanalytically oriented psychotherapy and behavior therapy seem very different, but they have certain things in common. Both fall under Wolberg's broad definition of psychotherapy, "a form of treatment for problems of an emotional nature in which a trained person deliberately establishes a professional relationship with the person with the object of removing, modifying, or retarding existing symptoms or mediating disturbed patterns of behavior and in promoting positive personality growth and development." [11] Although they have different immediate goals, the two therapies both ultimately work for happy, well-adjusted, symptom-free patients. Their strategies and specific methods certainly differ, as do the theories on which they rest.

But how important are specific methods and theories? The success of psychotherapy and behavior therapy might be due to some factor common to all therapies instead of, or even in spite of, their special techniques. Behavior therapists have argued that the successes of analytically oriented therapy are due to nondeliberate shaping of desired behavior. Many psychotherapists believe that behavior therapy succeeds only because of the trusting relationship that is incidentally formed between the behavior therapist and his patient. Rosenzweig has argued that

> Whether the therapist talks in terms of psychoanalysis or Christian Science is from this point of view relatively unimportant as compared with the *formal consistency* with which the doctrine employed is adhered to, for by virtue of this consistency the patient receives a schema for achieving some sort and degree of personality organization. [12]

In an effort to isolate the common factors of the two therapies which might produce success regardless of their theoretical frameworks, we measured the nature of the therapeutic relationship on several different dimensions. We also asked both therapists and patients for detailed descriptions of the important factors in their treatment.

# 2 How Psychotherapy Has Been Studied

Several reviews of the psychotherapeutic research literature are indispensable. Strupp and Bergin's excellent one provides a good feeling for the "state of the art" in 1969.[1] It includes detailed suggestions of goals and methodological standards for further research. The authors were optimistic that collaborative research would offer a significant new potential for resolving the dilemmas in the field. In particular this might apply to the problem of outcome which occupied only a small proportion of their vast bibliography of over two thousand references.[2]

The challenge of the outcome controversy was immediately answered by Meltzoff and Kornreich.[3] They analyzed 101 controlled outcome studies of psychotherapy, and were not led "convincingly to a conclusion in support of the null hypothesis." They considered that, in general, the better the quality of the research, the more positive the results obtained. They included all studies in which there was some kind of control sample and in which any kind of verbal therapy was used with any kind of patient. However, this extreme range of both therapies and patients, from hypnosis to "casual chats" with children, mental defectives, delinquents, alcoholics, and schizophrenics highlights Bergin's plea for specificity in outcome research.

In his superb review of the evaluation of therapeutic outcomes, Bergin emphasized the heterogeneous nature of reported studies, especially the diverse criteria of success.[4] These enabled Eysenck to establish idiosyncratic standards which permit three different views of the same case material, that of the original authors, Eysenck's, and a reader's own.[5] For example, dropouts are counted as failures by Eysenck, eliminated by Bergin, and might be more properly assigned by a third to success or failure, depending on their status at reassessment. In recognizing such methodological controversies Bergin paid belated tribute to Eysenck for arousing a dormant, if not moribund field. Eysenck himself has pointed more to his catalytic than to his seminal role. However, iconoclasts tend to be unloved.

Bergin made two more cardinal points. First, spontaneous remission in neurosis may be less than half the much quoted two-thirds. Second, in the 52 best controlled studies of neurosis there is a moderately positive average psychotherapeutic effect (22 positive, 15 doubtful, 15 negative). Not only was there no significant correlation between a study's outcome and its degree of control; there was even a slight tendency toward more positive outcome for studies with more rigorous designs (supporting Meltzoff and Kornreich). Most crucially, 53% of studies involving experienced therapists (20 out of 38) were positive, in contrast to 18% (2 out of 11) involving inexperienced therapists. However, experienced therapists accounted for 71% of negative outcomes, illustrating the "deterioration effects" in psychotherapy. Psychotherapy, while improving some patients, makes others worse. The fault may lie with the patient, the therapist, or an unhappy blend of the two. When the deterioration effects are added to the overall improvement rate of some two-thirds for all psychotherapy, Bergin concluded, there is *modest* evidence in favor of psychotherapy. In particular he cautioned that control for placebo effects has been poor.

The review of Luborsky *et al.* of factors influencing psychotherapeutic outcome is less extensive, but it is so concise and well organized that it can serve as an instant summary of the literature in any area.[6]

Finally, Malan's optimistic if not crusading review offers "renewed hope for the future."[7] As is the fashion, he reinterpreted Meltzoff and Kornreich's review, added an extra study by Orgel[8] and concluded that: (1) The evidence for the effectiveness of psychotherapy was relatively strong; (2) there was considerable evidence that dynamic psychotherapy was effective in psychosomatic conditions; but (3) the evidence in favor of dynamic psychotherapy in the ordinary run of neurosis and character disorders was weak in the extreme. However, he balanced this by his conviction, both from his own and the Menninger studies, that "meaningful outcome criteria correlated with meaningful variables which cannot be based on anything but clinical judgement . . . will save us in the future."[9] He believed that adequate research would find that particular psychoanalytic techniques would be appropriate for particular types of patients. Outcome would then be comparable to the description by Kessel and Hyman: "this patient was saved from an inferno and we are convinced that this could have been achieved by no other method."[10]

From the literature and from these cumulative reviews, one is struck by how remarkably few attempts were made until quite recently to explore the straightforward question, "Does psychotherapy do any good at all?" The skeptical observer is reminded of the director of a drug treatment center who was recently asked why he kept no statistics of any kind, and replied, "We like to think that we help *all* of our patients here, and I think it's better if we go on thinking so." [11] Besides this natural reluctance to question the general value of one's lifework, there are genuine difficulties involved in assessing therapeutic outcome.

The main problem is identifying standards of improvement and devising methods of measuring change. This is problem enough for a treatment like behavior therapy, whose stated goal is the removal of symptoms. It becomes Kafka-like for analytic therapies with such goals as the removal of unconscious conflicts, which by definition are imperceptible to begin with.

A second problem is that of control groups. No definite statement can be made about a treatment's effectiveness without some idea of how similar patients would fare without the treatment. But a therapist personally convinced of his treatment's worth naturally feels ethical qualms about depriving any patient of it for merely investigative reasons.

Third is the question of who shall measure progress. Both the therapist and the patient may have reasons for wanting the results to come out one way or the other but to provide independent assessors is expensive and time-consuming and to keep them blind to what treatment the patient has had is nearly impossible.

Fiske and his colleagues lucidly and comprehensively covered the minimum standards for research into the effectiveness of psychotherapy. [12] They pointed to the difficulty of attempting to evaluate psychotherapy:

> a treatment modality which has not been defined, the effects of which are presumed to require a long period of treatment, and the evaluation of which demands long-term follow-up. Furthermore,

> the treatment procedures are designed to modify conditions where the spontaneous recovery rate is considerable and the means of evaluating recovery controversial. Even fairly strong treatment effects might therefore easily be swamped by the heterogeneity of subject populations and the inevitable effects of intercurrent changes in life situations.

There has been increasing sophistication in the recommended criteria for measuring outcome of psychotherapy. Meehl merely pleaded for the use of control and experimental groups, pre- and post-therapy evaluation, and an adequate follow-up.[13] Eysenck listed introspective reports by the patient; observations of the patient by the therapist, an independent assessor, family, and friends; personality tests; physiological measures of the autonomic nervous system; and social action effects such as the number of arrests subsequent to treatment.[14]

Unfortunately, these recommendations have rarely been followed. Control groups have seldom been used, assessments have generally been done by the therapist or the patient with no other rater, follow-ups have been rare, and criteria for improvement have often not been explicitly stated. Direct replications are almost unknown, and each study has tested a slightly different hypothesis with idiosyncratic measures of outcome. Such practices inhibit the production of a coherent body of information about the effects of psychotherapy.

Sells, in pleading for more intelligent use of criteria, measurement, and control in psychotherapy research, quotes a charming story, illustrating what can happen when the researcher prefers his own judgment to that indicated by objective information.

> A few years ago I was impressed by an account of the method used to weigh pigs in Patagonia. In that country the pig was indispensable to the national economy as a source of food, leather, fats, and many by-products, and its weight a basic unit of exchange.

> Hence by regal decree it was required that pigs be weighed only at Government weighing stations by properly qualified and appointed weighmasters. At each weighing station a staff consisting of a supervisory master and four assistants, usually ranging from GS-9 to GS-13, would work as a team. Weighing was accomplished by means of a six-ply mahogany board, exactly 117 inches long and 29 inches wide, balanced on a tubular mahogany rod suspended between two uprights . . . When a pig was to be weighed, the board was first suspended on the rod and its position adjusted until it was in perfect balance . . . The pig was then placed in a marked-off space at one end of the board by the junior weighmasters while the others proceeded with the weighing process. From a case containing a wide variety of native rocks, ranging widely in size and shape but all highly polished and carefully smoothed, they would select one at a time and place each in neat rows beginning at the opposite end. Rocks were added and adjusted until the weight of the rocks exactly balanced the weight of the pig. The pig was then removed and the weighmasters would determine his weight. They would do this by counting the number of rocks of various sizes and shapes and converting their impressions into a global judgment expressed in terms of an average pig as a final weight.[15]

Investigators who have tried to measure psychotherapeutic outcome have taken different ways out of the dilemmas of criteria, measurement, and control, and their results are often therefore not directly comparable. Yet it is impressive how frequently an improvement rate of about two-thirds, *either with or without therapy*, is reported for neuroses, personality disorders, and other moderately severe problems typically seen in outpatients or in private office patients. Eysenck devoted considerable care to translating the diverse improvement criteria of 24 different outcome studies, and found 65% of patients remaining in treatment to be "improved."[16] He quoted similar figures for recovery without treatment reported by Landis[17] for severely neurotic inpatients receiving custodial care but little or no therapy, and by Denker[18] for individuals receiving insurance payments for neurotic disability, but no therapy.

This Landis-Denker-Eysenck baseline of "spontaneous" improvement, as Bergin has pointed out, has been macerated by criticism and cross-criticism.[19] Almost everyone agrees to the major deficiencies in the original samples and their interpretation, but no one has produced more accurate figures until Bergin's own reanalysis of 14 studies on "neurosis." In these, mostly recent and reasonably well controlled, Bergin deduced a median rate of improvement without therapy in the vicinity of 30%. This percentage he considered as perhaps unrealistically low and because of errors of measurement possibly as high as a median of 45%. It is characteristic of the field that he was soon attacked by Rachman who, reanalyzing some of the studies Bergin reviewed, raised the figure of spontaneous improvement about to where Bergin thought it might be anyway.[20] It would be more critical to reject delinquency, colitis, and peptic ulcer as "neurosis." These studies heavily skewed Bergin's figures. Similarly not everybody would accept the reported lengthy duration of symptoms before psychotherapy as a valid criterion of zero spontaneous improvement.

Part of the problem lies in the fact that the prognosis is bleaker for more serious problems. Goodwin[21] found only one-third of more severely disturbed inpatient obsessionals to be improved at a five-year follow-up, and Errera and Coleman[22] found that of 19 adult phobic patients contacted 23 years after treatment, 15 were still phobic.

In contrast, Schorer found that 65% of untreated neurotic outpatients on a waiting list had improved 5 years later, compared with 78% of treated patients from the same group.[23] This difference was not significant. Barron and Leary found no significant differences in the amount of MMPI improvement between neurotics who did, and neurotics who did not, receive psychotherapy.[24] Goodwin found that 60 to 70% of relatively mild obsessional outpatients were asymptomatic or improved after 5 years.[25] Amid all these conflicting figures of spontaneous improvement there is a further confounding factor in the often ignored "naturalistic" therapy from the many nonprofessional helping agents in society, which is emphasized in Bergin.[26]

Before considering improvement rates for different therapies, it must again be emphasized that results of different studies usually cannot be compared because of differences in criteria and method. For a variety of understandable reasons psychoanalysts have seldom published outcome studies.

Schlesinger has pointed out that

> Psychoanalysis has a long and troubled ambivalent attitude to research . . . [and] generally has seemed to feel defensive in regard to its place amongst the sciences. Challenges about the general validity of its findings lead inevitably to complaints about the scientific limitations of the private, secluded situation in which its findings are obtained, a situation that admits of no outside observers and seems in essence nonreplicable. Psychoanalysis has usually had to resort to explanations about the special nature of the two-party analytic situation, the necessity for confidentiality, and the impossibility of understanding what goes on in it by anyone who has not experienced it himself . . . until recently at least, such research was deemed to be unnecessary, even impossible . . . Anyone foolhardy enough to have proposed that what psychoanalysis needed was research into the psychoanalytic process would in all likelihood have been met by an effort to understand, sympathetically, the reasons for his 'doubts about psychoanalysis,' for which that sovereign remedy, 'more analysis,' was probably needed. At the same time, it has been said that every analyst is doing research when he is closeted with his patient, for isn't every analysis actually an experiment? Why, then, the need to import such alien concerns for measurement, validity, reliability, and bias, and to get involved in tortuous discussions of methodology?[27]

Schlesinger felt that his illustration approached caricature but that he had captured the prevailing climate of opinion. This climate has probably led to most of the studies extant being more or less "insight psychotherapy" or "psychoanalytically oriented therapy" rather than psychoanalysis. He concluded, and rightly, that if research in psychoanalysis is to be done it must be done by psychoanalysts themselves.

In fact, a Central Fact-Gathering Committee was formed in 1952 by the American Psychoanalytic Association. The Committee's sad history illustrates how elusive were the facts that it sought to gather. It was difficult for analysts to complete questionnaires. Ambiguities of diagnosis, nomenclature, and judgments of the effectiveness of treatment led to discouragement and an even lesser number of completed questionnaires. As a result, in 1957 the Committee was dissolved, another new committee was eventually appointed and in turn dissolved, and finally yet a third in 1961.

Six years later this last committee, under the chairmanship of Hamburg, bravely published the summarized findings. [28] Their paper is poignant with lost data and opportunity, but the picture is familiar to anyone who has attempted to study psychotherapy. Only 3,019 of the original total sample of 10,000 patients were still available for analysis. All these had both initial and terminal reports, since those with only initial reports had been lost. There was no way to compare the existing sample with the original one. The patients were heavily skewed toward better educated professional people, earning well. Many did not complete treatment. Of the 2,983 whose reports were examined, 43% were in psychoanalysis, 47% in psychotherapy, and 10% in both at different times. Of those in psychoanalysis 57% completed treatment as compared to 37% in psychotherapy and 47% in combined treatment. The more highly educated were more likely to complete treatment. There was no information in the study as to whether termination was initiated by the therapist or by the patient. Some of the results were as follows:

1. Depressed male patients showed 45.8% symptom cure as compared to 9% of the schizophrenic ones ($p<.001$). The overall symptom cure of 27% was surprisingly low. There was no significant relationship between age or income and cure.

2. Ninety-seven (97.3) percent of both males and females were judged by their therapist to be improved in total functioning.

3. Ninety-seven (96.6) percent of the patients reported they felt benefited by their treatment.

4. Psychoanalysis was significantly ($p < .001$) more effective than psychotherapy in curing symptoms. However, the analysts had selected for each group those who in their estimation would be most suited to that modality. They assigned the more highly educated to analysis. Also there was a difference in the intensity and duration of treatment between the two groups. Psychoanalysis was also significantly ($p<.001$) more effective in improving character structure than psychotherapy.

In conclusion, the committee pleaded for a more moderately scaled, sharply focused inquiry, which would permit greater specification for each variable and facilitate checks on the extent of interobserver agreement in coding each variable. They seemed to be somewhat disenchanted with the broad-scale pooling of information they had inherited and with the inconclusiveness of the results.

Rachman reviewed a number of further studies.[29] He concluded that there was no acceptable evidence to support the view that psychoanalytic treatment was effective. He quoted Bieber's study of homosexuality in which 19% (14 out of 72) of those who began treatment as exclusively homosexual eventually became heterosexual.[30] Only 7% of those patients who had fewer than 150 hours of treatment became heterosexual, in contrast to 47% of those who had more than 350 hours. Barendregt reported on patients who had psychological tests when they first applied for psychotherapy and then 2½ years later.[31] Forty-seven of these had been given psychoanalysis, 79 psychotherapy, and 74 had not had any form of psychotherapy or therapeutic contact. However, Rachman criticized the lack of randomization in the assignment to groups, the poor choice of criteria of change (including two projective tests of doubtful validity), and the fact that the psychoanalytic treatment was carried out predominantly by inexperienced psychoanalysts. In any case, results of the study did not yield evidence in favor of the therapeutic usefulness of either psychoanalysis or psychotherapy.

Seventy-six percent of a group of 30 patients studied by Klein regarded themselves as considerably improved after they had completed a minimum of 200 analytic sessions given 4 to 5 times weekly.[32] The psychoanalytic raters agreed with the patients but none of the ratings were made in a blind way. The Cremerius study[33] was reviewed by Eysenck[34] and re-reviewed by Rachman.[35] This was an 8 to 10 year follow-up after termination of treatment of 605 neurotic outpatients. There was little difference between the varieties of treatment at termination. At the follow-up there was a smaller deterioration in the patients who had received psychoanalytic psychotherapy as contrasted to verbal discussion, hypnosis, autogenic training, or combined methods. Psychoanalytic psychotherapy showed abolition of symptoms in 21% at this time compared to 41% at the end of treatment. This was significantly different from hypnosis where the figures were respectively 7 and 54%. However, those who had received psychoanalytic treatment had far more sessions, approximately

300 hours as opposed to a dozen hours or less for some of the other groups.

Eysenck's own review quoted five psychoanalytic studies whose improvement rates, ranging from 39% to 67%, averaged 44% but jumped to 66% when only those patients were considered who had finished their courses of therapy.[36] Weber *et al.* gave psychoanalytically oriented psychotherapy to 732 outpatients and found only 25% improved, according to ratings of their clinic records by independent judges.[37] Koegler and Brill found that neurotic patients who received an average of five months of analytically oriented therapy improved more than untreated or placebo patients on several scales, especially on scales rated by their therapists.[38] But at a two-year follow-up a psychiatric social worker found no differences remaining between the treated and untreated groups. Cappon found 75% of his own private neurotic outpatients improved at the end of Jungian-oriented therapy.[39] Rosenbaum found 70% of neurotic psychotherapy outpatients, preselected for good prognosis, much improved after a year.[40]

One of the best studies examining the outcome of treatment in terms of the underlying theory was conducted by Malan and his associates.[41] A psychoanalytic formulation of the patient provided an explanation of his neurotic symptoms. Criteria were established for a true, partial, or false resolution of the problem. For a true resolution, neurotic symptoms were required to disappear and the quality of interpersonal relationships, especially with heterosexual peers and authority figures, to improve. For partial resolution, substantial improvement in relationships without improvement in the neurotic symptoms, or limited improvement in both was required. Finally, a false resolution would result in loss of neurotic symptoms but there would be an accompanying withdrawal from human relationships. Of the 23 patients Malan and colleagues studied, they found 6 in the favorable and 3 in the partial or false resolution category, and 9 unchanged.

In a subsequent controlled study of 30 patients Malan confirmed the importance of the "transference-parent link" to good outcome.[42] He describes this as the therapist's emphasis on linking the transference relationship to the patient's relationships to his parents in childhood. This finding not only confirmed a long-standing principle of psychoanalytic therapy but extended its validity and allowed its application to brief psychotherapy. Similarly the Menninger Clinic immediately began to use their finding that supportive therapy was less effective for borderline patients than working through the transference relationship. Malan concluded, and he may well be right, that the main reason for the lack of research impact on clinical practice is the failure to design outcome criteria that do justice to the complexity of the human personality.

Partly because of their scientific, empirical orientation, behavior therapists have been far more willing than psychoanalysts to report outcome data. London has praised this rare virtue in the psychotherapy business while criticizing the inconclusiveness of much of their data.[43] Nevertheless, Eysenck, self-confessedly biased toward this discipline, has himself agreed that behavior therapists have not done conspicuously better than psychotherapists and psychoanalysts in demonstrating the clinical effectiveness of their methods. He adduces certain reasons why this might be so.[44] These involve the lack of comparability of patients, outcome criteria, and so forth, which plague the field.

Almost twenty years ago, using a variety of behavioral techniques, Wolpe reported a 90% improvement rate according to Knight's criteria (80 to 100% symptomatic improvement) with a group of 210 mixed neurotic patients.[45] Only one of 45 patients had relapsed when contacted several years later. A decade ago Lazarus reported an improvement rate of 78% in 408 neurotic patients.[46] Even with 126 patients with extremely severe neurosis and with an average of only 14 sessions of behavior therapy, he still managed an improvement rate of 62%. He found practically no symptom substitution or relapse after more than two years. Stampfl reported a cure rate of 100% for neurotic patients with his implosion therapy.[47]

Saper gives brief descriptions of 8 outpatients with various long-standing sexual, compulsive, and phobic disorders, all of whom had previously found some form of psychiatric treatment ineffective.[48] Six of these dramatically improved with behavior therapy techniques, primarily operant conditioning and systematic desensitization. Rachman, Hodgson, and Marks, treated 10 patients at least moderately handicapped by a chronic obsessive-compulsive disorder.[49] Six of these improved substantially or dramatically with short-term behavior therapy using either modelling or flooding, and this improvement persisted to follow-up three months later. These treatments were significantly more effective than a relaxation control treatment had been with these same patients. Hussain reported, but did not substantiate, a recovery rate of 95% of a group of 105 neurotic patients, using what he described as Wolpe's techniques.[50]

These studies, like most in the psychotherapy field, suffer some or all of the multiple defects of lack of control which we have already discussed. Without such control, we have no firm evidence of the general effectiveness of the psychotherapies or of the superior effectiveness of one form of therapy over another. Fortunately, in the last decade this problem has been increasingly tackled.

## TYPE OF THERAPY

A few studies have found evidence of significant improvement with psychotherapy, and significant differences in outcome between different types of therapy. Chief among these are two fairly recent, well-designed, and well-controlled ones: Paul's comparison[51] of insight therapy and desensitization for public speaking anxiety, and DiLoreto's [52] comparison of desensitization, client-centered, and rational-emotive therapy for interpersonal anxiety.

Paul's subjects were 96 undergraduates, enrolled in a required public speaking course, who had scored high on performance anxiety scales and had accepted an offer for free treatment for this anxiety. This treatment was provided by five experienced therapists, all with an "insight" orientation, either psychoanalytic or client-centered. These therapists were trained in the other two active treatments used in the study, and each used each of the three treatments.

Each subject in the active-treatment groups received five sessions of individual therapy. All therapists understood that reduction of performance anxiety was the criterion of success for all the treatments. A no-contact control group was unaware of its participation in the research, and merely took the pre- and post-treatment test batteries as did the entire class. Other subjects were assigned randomly to one of four other groups as follows.

1. Insight-oriented psychotherapy, consisting of the techniques ordinarily used by the therapists, attempted to reduce anxiety by helping the patient gain insight into the basis and interrelationships of his problem.

2. Wolpe's systematic desensitization, in slightly modified form, was given to the second group. The subject's history and current status were briefly explored and the things that made him most anxious when speaking in public were ranked. He received training in progressive relaxation and, while relaxed, visualized anxiety-arousing items of increasing impact. Therapists maintained a warm, interested, and helpful attitude, but discussion of dynamics was not permitted.

3. An attention-placebo procedure was given the third

group by the same therapists. This determined the extent of improvement from nonspecific treatment effects such as expectation of help, warmth, attention, and interest of the therapist, and suggestion and "faith." Subjects in this group could talk only briefly to the therapists about their problems. Most of the time in each session was devoted to a complicated procedure in which subjects were first given a "fast-acting tranquilizer," a 2-gram capsule of sodium bicarbonate. They were then, with great scientific rigmarole, asked to perform a boring task (discriminating among sonar signals on a recorded tape) which they were told was ordinarily a very stressful and anxiety-inducing task, but which would cause them no anxiety because of the tranquilizer they had taken. With repeated practice, they would gradually develop a tolerance for stress so that they would no longer become anxious in other stressful situations, even without the "tranquilizer."

4. A no-treatment control group followed the same procedures as the treatment groups, except for treatment itself. It differed from the no-contact group in that its members received a telephone call and a short interview from the experimenter, participated in two test speeches (in addition to those given by all students in the course) and were promised treatment sometime in the future, when a therapist would "become available."

After their second classroom speech, subjects in all but the no-contact control group gave a pretreatment test speech in groups of six to thirteen subjects. Each subject's audience consisted of the other subjects in that group plus four observers, advanced graduate students in clinical psychology who had been trained together (until their interobserver reliability exceeded .95), at rating the incidence of twenty behaviors indicative of anxiety, including hand tremors, perspiration, and voice quivers. Within a week of treatment termination, these same subjects all gave a similar post-treatment test speech. The pre- and post-treatment batteries administered to all students in the course included an anxiety differential; the IPAT Anxiety Scale Questionnaire; the Pittsburgh Social Extroversion-Introversion and Emotionality scales; four Interpersonal Anxiety scales ("speech before a large group," "competitive contest," "job interview," "final course examination") from the S-R Inventory of Anxiousness; and a short form of the "personal report of confidence as a speaker." Improvement on the various measures is summarized as follows:

1. The no-treatment control group did not improve significantly on any of the stress condition measures. These included an anxiety differential administered four minutes before the subject gave his pre- and post-treatment speeches, the subject's pulse rate taken one and a half minutes before his speech began, a palmar sweat index taken during the thirty seconds before his speech began, and the average of the observers' ratings of clinical manifestations of anxiety.

All three treated groups improved significantly, and significantly more than the no-treatment control group, on observable behavior and on anxiety as reported on the anxiety differential. On both these measures the systematic desensitization group improved significantly more than either the insight or the attention-placebo groups. Only the systematic desensitization group improved significantly on the two physiological measures. On *none* of these measures was there any significant difference between the insight and the attention-placebo groups. One group improved slightly more on some of the measures, the other group on the others.

2. The two performance-anxiety scales on the follow-up battery showed different patterns of significance, but in general results indicated that systematic desensitization had produced more improvement than the other two active

treatments, which were in turn more successful than the two control groups.

3. On the personality and anxiety scales of the follow-up battery, no group showed significant improvement on the anxiety differential or on emotionality. All four contact groups significantly shifted in the direction of extraversion on the Pittsburgh Social Extraversion-Introversion scale, with no significant intergroup differences in amount of improvement. Only on the IPAT scale of general anxiety were there significant intergroup differences. Both desensitization and the attention-placebo groups improved significantly more than the no-contact control group.

4. Self-ratings of improvement showed that subjects in all three formally treated groups felt they had benefited from treatment. The type of treatment had no significant effect on the degree of improvement they reported.

5. Therapists' ratings indicated that, in their judgment, subjects in the systematic-desensitization group improved significantly more than both other treated groups on performance anxiety. The attention-placebo group improved significantly more than the insight group. However, the therapists rated the insight group as having improved significantly more than the other groups in areas other than performance anxiety. This result was not substantiated by any of the other measures and may reflect the therapists' bias in favor of insight therapy. This seems unlikely, however, since the therapists indicated after treatment that desensitization, or desensitization-plus-insight would have been the most appropriate treatment in the majority of cases.

Paul's conclusion, then, was that systematic desensitization was most effective. On some measures it was effective with 100% of subjects. He also found that, at least on a short-term basis, the nonspecific factors of relationship, attention, and suggestion produce as much anxiety reduction as gaining "insight" and "self-understanding." Moreover, the advantage of systematic desensitization was maintained over time.

Two years after treatment Paul obtained, by mail, follow-up information from all his treated subjects and from 70% of his control patients, an astonishingly high return considering the high mobility of the sample.[53] On most measures, improvement was not only maintained but also increased. At this point there were still no significant differences between the insight and attention-placebo groups, although both still showed significantly greater treatment effects than the control groups. The systematic desensitization group was still significantly more improved than all other groups. On a composite of all the speech-anxiety scales, significant improvement from initial assessment was shown by 85% of the desensitization patients, 50% each of the insight and attention-placebo patients, and 22% of the controls.

Paul concluded that his results

> clearly demonstrate the superiority of treatment based on a 'learning' model (modified systematic desensitization) over treatment based on the traditional 'disease' model (insight-oriented psychotherapy) in the alleviation of maladaptive anxiety . . . In general we may conclude that the majority of cases currently seen in clinics and counseling bureaus, especially those in which anxiety is a prominent problem, may be treated effectively by re-educative procedures in a relatively short period of time.

Certainly Paul's results are often cited as evidence of the superiority of behavior therapies, and to some extent this is justified. Clearly desensitization was superior in this instance. Such a clearcut result is impressive in a study with excellent experimental design and controls, which used experienced therapists and diverse but relevant measures of outcome. In view of the quality of this investigation, its results can probably be generalized to other, similar situations; unfortunately there is doubt whether they can be generalized to more common clinical situations.

The most serious problem with Paul's study is that its subjects were not actual patients but volunteers who were solicited for research. He emphasizes that in most of his patients anxiety was not restricted to the speech situation but was present in almost any social, interpersonal, or evaluative situation, and he lists many symptoms of anxiety reported by these students. Nevertheless, the subjects had not sought therapy for these other areas of anxiety. In fact, there was little evidence that the desensitization had affected the other areas. Nor had the patients actively sought treatment for their speech performance anxiety; they accepted it only when it was persuasively offered them. It seems likely that these subjects differed in motivation for treatment from the more usual psychotherapeutic patients. They also probably suffered less distress and incapacity, from problems that were not so pervasive and complex. We cannot know to what extent these differences hold, so we cannot know to what degree Paul's results can be applied to more general therapeutic situations.

Although DiLoreto's subjects were also recruited from a class (in this case a large introductory psychology class), this criticism is somewhat less applicable to his study since students were accepted who suffered from high self-reported interpersonal or social anxiety of any sort. One hundred students who wished to accept an offer of free treatment, and who scored high on DiLoreto's interpersonal anxiety scale, were randomly assigned to one of five treatment groups. Therapists in the active-treatment groups were six advanced graduate students in counseling and clinical psychology, who had had supervised training and at least one year of practical experience in their respective techniques. All actively-treated subjects received nine hours of group therapy; each therapist treated two groups of five subjects each.

The three actively-treated groups received rational-emotive therapy, client-centered therapy, and systematic desensitization. A no-treatment control group attended first, last, and follow-up group sessions in which each subject's history and problem were briefly explored so that behavior ratings of interpersonal anxiety could be made. However, no direct therapy took place. This group was promised treatment beginning at the end of the school term. In addition, the author met with them in five-person subgroups for lunch three times during the period in which other groups were receiving therapy. These control groups discussed academic problems, educational matters, and midterm examinations. No formal therapy took place, but the author attempted to maintain good rapport by expressing concern, understanding, and tolerance.

The no-contact control group did not receive behavior ratings. They took the pre-test battery with the other subjects and met all selection criteria, but were never contacted for treatment and were thus unaware of their participation in the study. Post-test and follow-up batteries were obtained from these subjects by mail.

Measures of improvement included a battery of tests given before therapy began, after therapy ended, and three months after the completion of therapy. At each therapy session, subjects completed a State Anxiety Inventory and submitted an index of interpersonal activity recording the nature and extent of such activity during the preceding week. Therapists then completed a rating sheet, estimating the degree of each subject's anxiety during that session. Finally, two trained and highly reliable raters observed and recorded behaviors indicative of anxiety during the first therapy session; during a post-therapy evaluation session, and during a follow-up meeting three months later. In the post-therapy evaluation, the groups were reorganized so that no subject was in a group with the counselor or with any of the other subjects who had been in his treatment group. This was true also of the follow-up group meeting three months later, for which the groups were again entirely reorganized. These meetings with strangers were felt to be situations of interpersonal stress.

Results at the end of treatment may be summarized as follows.

First, on a self-rating scale of interpersonal anxiety, on the behavioral ratings of interpersonal anxiety, and on "general anxiety" as measured by the S-R inventory of anxiousness, all the treatments had produced significantly more improvement than either of the control conditions. On these measures, the systematic desensitization subjects improved significantly more than the rational-emotive or client-centered subjects.

Second, the rational-emotive treatment produced the greatest increase in interpersonal activity outside the treatment setting. The increase was significantly more than that produced by systematic desensitization, which, in turn, was significantly more than that produced in subjects who received either client-centered or placebo treatment.

Third, this general pattern of improvement was maintained over time. At the three-month follow-up, subjects who received the three treatments were all still significantly more improved than recipients of either of the control conditions, on all the behavior ratings and self-reports of interpersonal and general anxiety. Similarly, the systematic desensitization group had maintained the significance of its advantage over the client-centered and rational-emotive groups.

Fourth, some nonspecific effect of therapy (such as the counselor's warmth and interest, or the subject's expectation of help) certainly obtained. The no-treatment (placebo) condition was significantly more effective in reducing self-reports of anxiety than the no-contact control condition, both at completion of treatment and at three-month follow-up.

Finally, the various treatments had different effects on introverted and extraverted subjects, as distinguished by the Myers-Briggs type indicator. The client-centered and systematic-desensitization groups of extraverted subjects improved significantly more than the rational-emotive or either control group of extraverted subjects on the various measures of interpersonal and general anxiety, and this difference was maintained at follow-up. There was no significant difference among any of the groups of extraverted subjects in terms of changes in interpersonal activity outside of treatment.

In contrast, among introverted subjects the rational-emotive and systematic desensitization treatments produced (and maintained until follow-up) significantly more improvement than the client-centered and control conditions. The client-centered subjects showed significantly more improvement than the no-contact group, but not more than the no-treatment control groups. Thus the overwhelming general success of systematic desensitization could be at least partially attributed to the fact that *it worked equally well with introverts and extraverts*, while extraverts treated with rational-emotive therapy and introverts treated with client-centered therapy improved no more than their placebo-treated counterparts. DiLoreto discusses this fact in the light of the theories underlying the three therapies.

DiLoreto's excellent study, which demonstrates the superiority of desensitization as clearly as does Paul's, shares to a limited extent the latter's major flaw, the use of solicited subjects rather than "real patients." DiLoreto's subjects probably more nearly resemble real patients, since they suffered from and were treated for more generalized interpersonal anxiety than were Paul's; nevertheless they had not themselves actively sought therapy, and it is hard to compare their motivation or need for treatment, or the complexity of their problems, with those of actual patients.

A more serious flaw is DiLoreto's use of relatively inexperienced therapists. The two client-centered therapists had sharply different success rates, as did the two rational-emotive therapists, and in each case the more successful therapist had nearly twice as much experience as his less successful colleague. Each therapist treated one group of extraverts and one group of introverts, so that counselor effects were not simply confounded with personality-type effects. The client-centered counselors were both equally effective with extraverts (which may be thought of as their "easy" patients) and the rational-emotive therapists were both equally effective with their introverts. But with "difficult" clients in each therapy, the more experienced therapist was significantly more effective than his less experienced colleague.

The two behavior therapists were about equally effective with introverts and extraverts. Evidence is cited later in this chapter that less experience may be required to attain some minimal level of competence with behavior therapy than with other forms of psychotherapy (see notes 78 and 79). Since none of these therapists had extensive experience, and since experience was clearly a factor in the success of the nonbehavioral therapists, it may be that DiLoreto was comparing the effectiveness of therapists who had attained very different degrees of the expertise required for the success of their respective treatments.

A few other studies have found significant differences in outcome between different kinds of therapy. Stone, Imber, and their colleagues compared patients who received minimal contact therapy or analytically oriented group or individual therapy.[54] They found that at six months patients with the most therapeutic contact had improved most in "social effectiveness" (but not in degree of discomfort or other measures) and that this effect had disappeared at five-year follow-up. Land found relatively directive group therapy more effective with chronic, very withdrawn inpatients, and extremely nonactive therapy more effective with more active, less deteriorated patients.[55] Straker, working with outpatients, found more directive, symptom-oriented therapy to be far more successful and with a far lower dropout rate than longer term, more analytic therapy.[56] Schofield found that the MMPI's of hospitalized neurotics improved significantly after a month in hospital, while outpatient neurotics' MMPI's did not improve after a month (five sessions) in therapy.[57,58] There are many other such solitary results but no coherent body of research in any one area, except for a small body of research comparing the results of behavior therapy and insight-oriented psychotherapy.

Gelder, Marks, and Wolff found that severely phobic patients recovered faster with behavior therapy than with either individual or group psychotherapy, but after all treatment was complete the results of behavior therapy were no longer significantly better.[59] In another study by this group, matched patients receiving behavior therapy and individual psychotherapy had equal improvement rates.[60] In still others, results were mixed, with behavior therapy patients generally showing more improvement in certain areas than patients who did not receive either behavior therapy or any other consistent therapy.[61,62,63] But these differences were no longer significant at follow-up. In these studies patients were often given other treatments, including drugs, simultaneously with the therapies whose effects were being studied. Also they were often not assigned randomly to treatment, that is, they might be assigned to the desensitization group after long courses of other treatments had failed.

Marks and Gelder also share the near-universal limitation of behavior therapy studies, that of treating only phobics, compulsives, and others with "unitary" problems. This tendency is understandable, since change in a phobia is so much more easily measured than change in a less circumscribed anxiety neurosis and since phobias, especially, are thought to be especially susceptible to behavioral treatment. But it would be of more practical interest to know the results of behavior therapy with the anxiety neuroses and personality disorders which are so much more common in average outpatient populations and private patients, at least in this country.

The same caveat applies to several experiments attempting to identify the essential effective elements of behavior therapies, using volunteers with snake phobias as subjects. Bandura found that desensitization and vicarious modeling by watching a film substantially reduced phobic behavior as compared with a control group, but was less effective than live modeling and guided participation, which eliminated the phobia in nearly all patients.[64] Also using snake phobics, Leitenberg[65] found praise and induction of favorable expectation to be very important to outcome, and Davison[66] showed that both relaxation and a graded hierarchy of phobically relevant images were important and needed to be paired in order to obtain a satisfactory outcome. Such studies are scientifically important and illustrate the interest in the mechanism of change which has been characteristic of recent behavior therapy studies, but their fantastically high improvement rates (often nearly 100% cure) cannot be taken at face value. Although subjects must meet standards of avoidance behavior in order to be used in these studies, most are far from being real phobics in the usual sense of the word.

## THERAPIST VARIABLES

Although "personality" and "style" of either therapist or patient are difficult to define and measure, they are continually being defined and measured in different terms. Not surprisingly the findings are seldom replicated, seldom believed, and almost never applied in clinical practice. They nevertheless cover a wide field.

The ideal therapist is described by Krasner as mature, well-adjusted, sympathetic, tolerant, patient, kindly, tactful, nonjudgmental, accepting, permissive, noncritical, warm, likeable, intelligent, and so on through several dozen laudatory adjectives.[67] He is no more believable than any other folk hero. There is little evidence that any of the standard personality tests can discriminate successful from unsuccessful therapists. Bergin and Jasper[68] and Frayn[69] found therapeutic skill unrelated to the therapist's scores on the MMPI and the Minnesota-Hartford Personality Assay, and Holt and Luborsky[70] found unreliable the previous tentative relationship they had observed between therapeutic success and therapist's T.A.T. scores. In the present study the Eysenck Personality Inventory was used as a measure of therapist extraversion-introversion and neuroticism.

A multitude of studies have been done on the A-B therapist variable developed from the Strong Vocational Interest Blank by Betz and Whitehorn.[71] A-type therapists have Strong scores similar to those of lawyers and accountants; B-types have scores like those of printers and science teachers. Razin[72] and Chartier[73] have critically reviewed this research, considering differential clinical outcome, personal characteristics, and analogue studies. Outcome studies found A's more effective with schizophrenics than B's, and B's more effective with neurotics.[74] The most recent data emphasize the importance of improvement criteria; A's seem more successful in relieving subjective distress and B's in effecting impulse control, especially with schizophrenics. Personal characteristics studies find A's more trusting, intropunitive, and tolerant of "inner" experiences and spontaneity, more field-dependent and personally involved with patients, and more oriented to problem solving than B's.

Analogue laboratory studies suggest that A's share with, and communicate to, schizophrenics an awareness of idiosyncratic perceptions and that they are able to inspire trust in such patients. Chartier argues that extensive laboratory research has failed to increase understanding of the original phenomena and that analogue studies constitute a premature simplification of an insufficiently understood interaction. The rash of simulated and in-therapy experiments is typical of the way preoccupation with process bedevils the field. Chartier urges the necessity for verifying A-B effects in a good naturalistic study of psychotherapy. There probably is some powerful factor involved, but only a minority of studies have used adequate outcome criteria. We administered the A-B scale to all therapists at the beginning of the present study, so that the A-B effect on patient outcome could be measured.

There is some evidence[75, 76] that experienced therapists generally have better results than novices and that patients prefer older therapists because of their apparent greater experience.[77] This may mean that unduly gloomy results have been obtained in that great majority of studies where the therapy has been done by residents, medical students, interns, counselling students, or other beginning therapists, in whose hands a treatment cannot be expected to achieve its full potential. There is also some suggestion that a shorter period of training is required for beginning behavior therapists than for beginning psychotherapists to attain some minimal level of competence.[78, 79] If that is true, we would have given an unfair advantage to behavior therapy had we used beginning therapists in this study. For both these reasons, only experienced therapists treated patients in this study. It was hoped that the use in each treatment group of therapists with differing amounts of experience might show some effect of experience on outcome. If so, it might confirm Fiedler's finding that, in their therapeutic relationships, expert therapists of different schools are more like one another than like nonexpert therapists of their own schools.[80]

## PATIENT AND PROBLEM VARIABLES

Most of the studies of patient variables have hinged on the patient's suitability for traditional, usually insight, psychotherapy, and have been even less systematic than studies of therapist variables. There is considerable evidence that therapists prefer patients of the opposite sex who are young, attractive, verbal, intelligent, and successful (the YAVIS syndrome of Schofield).[81, 82, 83] These patients apparently have better outcomes.[84] Even in clinics where ability to pay is not a factor, patients of higher socioeconomic status as compared to low are more likely to seek therapy, to be given it, and to remain in it for a substantial length of time.[85, 86, 87] This is also true of Caucasian as compared to non-Caucasian patients.[88] This is not to say that they improve more. Goldstein calls the selection process more of an exclusion one.[89] This works by a sort of fiat growing out of an admixture of clinical reports and therapeutic traditions, and excludes patients labeled psychopathic, sociopathic, delinquent, antisocial, unmotivated, unsuitable, nonverbal, or coerced into therapy against their will. It certainly excludes people who are not intelligent, of lower social class, or too sick. These assumptions deserve to be examined. We used the Mill Hill vocabulary scale as a measure of intelligence and collected complete demographic data on every patient, including age, sex, race, education, socioeconomic status, and religion, among others.

There have been scattered studies differentiating between successful and unsuccessful patients on the basis of Rorschach scores[90, 91] or MMPI scores. Harris, for example, found that successful patients had a concentration of high MMPI scores on hypochondriasis, hysteria, and depression, and a secondary peak at psychasthenia; that is, they were typically neurotic, in contrast with unsuccessful patients, who had higher psychopathic deviate, paranoia, schizophrenia, and mania scores.[92]

Studies relating outcome to the type of psychiatric problem have tended both to be idiosyncratic and to use mostly unreliable methods of measuring outcome. Usually, even with global diagnoses, there are not good studies to support clinical beliefs, although in general patients diagnosed as neurotic do better than those diagnosed as psychotic or personality or behavior disordered.[93, 94] Patients in this research took several personality inventories, including the MMPI, the Eysenck Personality Inventory, and part of the California Psychological Inventory. Outcome was measured against the results of these and against the patient's diagnosis and the severity of his illness.

Patients who have a considerable desire to do something about their problems often seem to do best. Certainly the patient's apparent motivation is important to the way his therapist sees him. Appel[95] and Tissenbaum[96] both found that therapists mentioned motivation for therapy most often when asked to list factors related to treatment outcome. Wallach and Strupp found that patients who were eager to seek and accept psychiatric help were perceived by psychotherapists as having greater ego strength, more anxiety, more insight into their problems, and more favorable prognoses than those they classified as having low motivation for therapy.[97] The therapist also felt warmer and more willing to accept highly motivated patients into treatment. Much of this perception may be a halo effect. Raskin found that patients whose therapists rated them as highly motivated were also more educated, had a higher occupational level, expected psychotherapy rather than physical or medical treatment, and were better liked and rated more psychologically aware by the therapist.[98] Strupp has summed this up as a general belief that the keys to successful psychotherapy include eagerness to help and willingness to work with another person, ability to withstand pain from emerging feelings during therapy, and a level of emotional maturity high enough to make this possible.[99] Malan endorses this capacity for insight from his own studies.[100]

Frank believes that the arousal of hope and the expectation of relief are important factors in any form of psychotherapy.[101] Stone *et al.* found in several studies that patients showed improved comfort and mood prior to beginning therapy, often after only one evaluation interview.[102] They also found that therapists who believed the patient would improve were more successful than therapists whose expectations were lower. It is an extremely difficult task to measure motivation or expectation of improvement, and we made no direct attempt to do so. The control group was randomly assigned from the same population as the treated patients, so presumably were equally motivated. They had a long assessment interview and the promise of eventual treatment, which probably provided some "arousal of hope" and other effects of an initial therapy session.

## PATIENT-THERAPIST INTERACTION

Similar studies relating outcome or length of therapy to similarity of patient-therapist personality have found positive,[103] negative,[104] curvilinear,[105] and nonexistent[106, 107] relationships between the two. Such research is problematical because of the difficulty of measuring personality, let alone personality similarity. Attempts to study the effects of similarity on such dimensions as socioeconomic status or education are confounded because the therapists are much alike. Any effects of the patient's similarity to the therapist could be more accurately ascribed to the patient's absolute level. For example, the patient might well be judged "well-educated" rather than "similar to therapist in educational level."

The therapist's behavior during the therapeutic interview is of great importance. Truax has isolated several variables on which a therapist can be rated with high reliability by trained raters listening to recordings of therapy sessions.[108] He found that patients who receive high levels of "empathy, warmth, and genuineness" from their therapists have significantly better outcomes than patients receiving low levels. Truax found that these variables were independent of one another, but others found high intercorrelations, suggesting the existence of a single "good-therapist" variable.[109] Nevertheless the correlation of good outcome with high levels of Truax variables (and with a similar set of variables developed by Lorr[110]) has been replicated several times. Although Truax himself has tested his variables with client-centered therapy, there seems no reason why these factors should be less important to other therapeutic relationships, and Truax ratings were made for one session with nearly every patient in the present research. Staples and Sloane have found that patients improve more the more time they spend talking (the less time the therapist spends talking) in the therapy sessions, and also that the longer the duration of the patient's average speech in therapy the more he improves.[111,112] We measured these and other "speech patterns" from transcripts of entire sessions between nearly every patient and his therapist.

## FEATURES OF THE PRESENT STUDY

The present research was designed after an exhaustive review of the literature. In summary, we considered the following features important in our study:

1. The use of experienced practitioners of behavior therapy and psychoanalytically oriented therapy.
2. A wait-list group where the minimal treatment involved in assessment, promise of treatment, and follow-up probably aroused hope and expectation of improvement. In addition, crisis care was easily available.
3. Random assignment of patients to psychoanalytically oriented therapy, behavior therapy, or wait-list.
4. The use of an independent assessment team who tried to make their follow-up assessments as nearly blind as possible and who resisted the temptation to analyze data until the last patient had been interviewed.
5. The use of typical patients who attended a university psychiatric outpatient clinic. They proved to be suffering from quite severe psychoneuroses or personality disorders which are usually considered amenable to psychotherapy.
6. An independent team to analyze data during and after the study.
7. Information from relatives or friends of the patient.
8. Multiple outcome measures; target symptoms and measures of overall function derived from therapist, patient, assessor, relative, and psychological tests.
9. Standardized procedures. Definition of target symptoms; Structured and Scaled Interview to Assess Maladjustment for work and social adjustment; MMPI, Eysenck Personality Inventory, California Psychological Inventory to assess kind and extent of pathology and its effect on outcome.
10. A check on in-therapy procedures to show both qual-

itative and quantitative differences among: treatments, therapists, patients, and therapist-patient interaction.

11. A follow-up at one year and two years from original assessment.

# 3 The Plan of the Study

This study had four major aims. The first was to compare the effectiveness of behavior therapy, analytically oriented psychotherapy and a minimal contact treatment.

The second aim was to examine the similarities and differences between behavior therapy and psychotherapy. At first glance the differences between these treatments seem great, but many of the distinctions blur on closer examination. There is considerable controversy as to the effective ingredients of psychotherapy and whether there are common elements in the two treatments which lead to the desired outcome, regardless of the theoretical orientation of the therapist. Acceptance into any kind of treatment arouses hope that tomorrow may be less bleak than today. This is an example of one of these common, nonspecific factors.

Certain variables tend to be more strongly emphasized by one school than by another. The quality of the patient-therapist relationship, for example, is considered critical to analytically oriented therapy, while behavior therapists consider this to be of minimal importance once a basic working relationship is established. We tried to investigate more precisely what behavior therapists and insight therapists actually do in their treatment, what the relationship is like in the two therapies, and what the patients and therapists of each group think about the treatment and each other.

Third, we intended to investigate the effect on outcome of the therapist's level of experience and of certain of his personality characteristics.

The fourth aim of the research was to investigate what kind of patients or problems yield to therapeutic intervention. That is, to determine whether patients with certain characteristics (e.g., sex, age, personality type) or certain kinds of problems are more likely to improve regardless of treatment. If treatment can be credited for their improvement, are they more amenable to treatment by behavior therapy than by insight therapy or vice versa? What treatment features might be responsible for this?

## PROCEDURE

In order to provide the unwary reader with a map of the swampy methodological terrain to follow, we present a brief overview of the plan of the study. Patients who were considered by experienced psychiatrists to be suitable candidates for a "talking-type" therapy were randomly assigned to one of three treatment conditions: a minimum of thirty each to behavior therapy, to analytically oriented psychotherapy, and to a minimal contact wait list. Three experienced therapists in each of the active treatment groups saw a minimum of ten patients each for up to four months.

All patients were seen individually by one of three psychiatric assessors at the initial assessment (before assignment to treatment), again four months later (after the controlled treatment period), and again one year after the initial assessment. At each of these assessments, measures of the severity of the patients' main target symptoms were taken along with a measure of general personality functioning, to be described. Patients were also seen two years after the initial assessment by a research assistant.

*Assessors*

The three assessors had received different kinds of psychiatric training and had differing interests.

Assessor X, a British-trained psychiatrist, emigrated to North America following his psychiatric residency. He had had a personal analysis and had treated neurotic patients along analytically oriented lines, but he was also interested in behavior therapy. He had himself treated 1,200 neurotic patients over a period of 22 years.

Assessor Y, an American-trained psychiatrist, had received a training which emphasized psychoanalytically oriented psychotherapy, He was enthusiastic about treating patients according to these principles, although he had not had a personal analysis. This assessor had treated 300 patients in 10 years, and he had occasionally used techniques of behavior modification in conjunction with his more usual insight methods.

Assessor Z, a British-trained psychiatrist, had also emigrated to the United States subsequent to his psychiatric training. His special interest was behavior modification based on application of the principles of Skinnerian learning theory. He was very critical of analytic psychotherapy, somewhat critical of behavior therapy, and tended to regard neurosis as a spontaneously remitting condition. He had treated 900 neurotic patients over the course of 19 years.

The fourth member of the assessment team was the research assistant, who prepared patients for their assessments, maintained telephone contact with patients on the waiting list, and at the time of each assessment interviewed a close friend or relative of the patient (the "informant") in order to obtain another viewpoint of his problems and progress. The assistant was a college graduate in her early 20's, with no formal graduate training but considerable psychological sophistication, and she was warm, friendly, and successful in putting patients at ease.

## MEASURES OF OUTCOME

The principal measures of treatment effectiveness were changes in the severity of three target symptoms, varying from one individual to another, and changes in general adjustment. Target symptom measurement and the SSIAM are described here. Other measures will be described later, as appropriate.

### *Target Symptoms*

Taking into account the wide range of problems for which our patients sought help, our main outcome measure was tailored to each patient's symptoms. During the first assessment interview the patient was encouraged to talk freely about his problems, his family, his background, and his life in general. When the assessor felt he understood the situation, he and the patient together identified the patient's three leading problems. Each was formulated in terms acceptable to the patient, which summarized the problem in such a way that change could be recognized.

The three target symptoms might obviously pertain to one central problem (impotence, worry over impotence, feelings of inferiority to other males) or might seem unrelated (compulsive eating, pulling out hair, apprehension with important people). The object of choosing individual symptoms was to allow the patient to define his problems and his goals in therapy rather than to set some universal standard that would necessarily be vague and that might be irrelevant to the patient's own reasons for seeking treatment. For example, there were several homosexual patients with such target symptoms as excessive smoking, feelings of unreality, uncontrollable temper, and excessive fatigue. Either they did not want to change their sexual orientation or else this was a relatively unimportant goal. If, with treatment, their sexual adjustment changed, this was taken into account in measures of happiness and of overall and specifically sexual adjustment. But their symptomatic improvement rating depended on the success of therapy in changing those symptoms they originally wanted changed.

The patient estimated when each target symptom first appeared, when he last experienced it, its average frequency and duration, and when he last felt at ease in that situation. These ratings served both to quantify distress and to give the assessor as precise an idea as possible of the problem's extent. After gathering all this information about a target symptom the psychiatrist made the global rating of severity: zero for absent, 1 for doubtful or trivial, 2 mild, 3 moderate, or 4 severe.

At each reassessment, the assessor again rated the severity of each target symptom, without refreshing his memory as to the initial severity. Improvement was defined as the difference between the initial and post-treatment severity of the symptoms. An originally severe (4) symptom which was mild (2) after four months' therapy was rated as 2 points' improvement.

In additon to ratings of absolute severity, from which change scores were calculated, the assessor also directly rated the amount of change he saw in a symptom since the original rating, and this was done on a 13-point scale ranging from "very much worse" (zero) through "no change" (6) to "completely recovered" (12).

### *Structured and Scaled Interview to Assess Maladjustment*

Although symptomatic improvement was the most important measure of patient change, it does not necessarily reflect changes in general adjustment which may make the patient much happier. A patient's symptoms might stubbornly remain while his work, his relationships, and his sexual life all dramatically improved. Or he might lose all his symptoms and still be generally miserable. Neither aspect of improvement can be ignored.

In order to measure changes in adjustment, a questionnaire called the Structured and Scaled Interview to Assess Maladjustment (SSIAM) was used.[1] Two SSIAM ratings were done simultaneously. While the assessor was interviewing the patient, the research assistant interviewed the relative or friend in a separate room to obtain a second set of SSIAM ratings for the patient. The SSIAM is a new and reliable method for measuring social maladjustment, which a trained interviewer can complete in about half an hour and which patients and relatives find relevant, thorough, and acceptable. It consists of ten items about each of five areas of adjustment: work, social, sexual, relations with family of origin, and relations with present family. Each item is rated on an eleven-point severity scale with five clearly defined anchor points. The SSIAM is described in detail in Appendix 1.

## CHOOSING THE PATIENTS

Previous psychotherapy studies have too often described the raw material of the therapeutic mix in rather vague terms such as "neurotic outpatients" or "psychiatric patients" with a passing reference to the range of ages and psychiatric diagnoses of the sample. To take seriously the problem of identifying more clearly the conditions under which change occurs in therapy requires a precise description of the characteristics of the patients treated.

### *Source of Referrals*

During the time of our investigation as many as possible of the patients of the Temple University Psychiatric Outpatient Clinic were screened for the study. These came from a variety of sources: the health services of nearby colleges, referrals from local hospitals without adequate psychiatric facilities, self-referrals, and the local community mental health center. Usually this assessment replaced that of the initial visit to the clinic which followed a telephone interview by the clinic's social worker. However, because the clinic was heavily committed to training medical students and residents, who normally assessed patients under supervision, some were referred after their initial assessment. A few had received brief psychotherapy (usually analytically oriented) by residents or students before being referred to the project for more intensive therapy.

With so many calls on the clinic for patients, we also experienced the syndrome so aptly described by Koegler and Brill as "the vanishing American." Hordes of patients demanding psychotherapy have a tendency to disappear like morning dew when you need them. The reason for this is twofold. Any research makes clinicians leery. The referring ones tend to refer elsewhere—the psychoanalysts because their patients might get behavior therapy, the behaviorists because they might get analytically oriented therapy, and both because their patients might have to wait four months. Of course there were built-in protections for the patient, and most psychotherapy clinics in the city had waiting lists longer than four months, but nevertheless the clinic staff saw ogres behind every protocol. They felt slighted by lack of consultation (despite endless talks) and frightened both by a possible lack of patients for their training programs and by a possible deluge of patients who would want more therapy after the project ended. The assessors guaranteed not to offend on any count. If there were insufficient patients for training, they would cut back; if there were too many off the end of the assembly line, they would treat them themselves or find someone to do it outside the clinic.

In the end all worked out happily, but communication between the research team and the clinic was perhaps the least successful aspect of the study. Despite housing in the clinic and close personal relationships, some of the clinic staff felt bruised by the research. The researchers in turn felt a mixture of *mea culpa* and self-righteous annoyance that their pure scientific efforts should be so misinterpreted.

### *Criteria for Acceptance*

An individual was a suitable subject for this study on the following counts: (1) if he was a psychiatric patient but not extremely severely disturbed, (2) if he wished to receive psychotherapy, (3) if psychotherapy was the treatment of choice for him in the opinion of the assessor, and (4) if he was between the ages of eighteen and forty-five. Twenty-nine applicants did not meet these requirements and were referred elsewhere or treated outside the boundaries of the study.

By the first criterion, a "psychiatric patient" was defined as one who felt subjective discomfort, whose symptoms interfered with his proper functioning in work, social, or sexual life, and who was prompted to seek psychiatric help for these difficulties.

At one extreme, this excluded relatively normal people who viewed therapy as more of an educational, broadening experience than as a treatment for real and specific emotional difficulties, and patients who were so vague as not to be able to articulate any tangible target problem. Seven patients were excluded for these reasons, and another five were not accepted because their problems reflected mild situational disturbances resulting from temporary conditions in their environment which were likely to change in the immediate future. At the other extreme, patients were excluded whose very severe problems either could not safely wait four months for help (potential suicides) or indicated a poor prognosis with any kind of short-term therapy (alcoholism, drug addiction, schizophrenia, organic brain damage, and sexual deviation, although a few homosexuals were accepted for treatment of other problems). One patient was excluded from the study because his brain had been damaged in an automobile accident.

Under the second criterion, a patient was accepted if he was willing and able to take part in four months of some kind of "talking therapy," and did not demand drugs or some other kind of treatment instead. Six patients were excluded because they planned to move from the area in less than four months. Another was unable to come at a reasonable time, one refused therapy altogether, and one began treatment with another psychiatrist after the initial contact.

The assessor accepted, by the third criterion, only those patients whom he would himself under ordinary circumstances have accepted or referred for psychotherapy rather than for any other treatment. Five patients were excluded on this basis, most of them with severe depressions for which antidepressant drugs were more appropriate treatments.

Patients under 18 were excluded because their rapid changes in growth and maturity often have beneficial effects that are difficult to separate from those caused by therapy. Patients over 45 are less often candidates for therapy and are more likely to be suffering either from affective disorders or from situational factors much less amenable to therapy than those of younger adulthood and early middle age. Two patients were excluded for reasons of age: a man of 63 and a woman of 69.

Evelyn Ashley was rather typical of the patients accepted for treatment. A pale, sullen-looking college senior who chain-smoked cigarettes, she had since the age of four withdrawn from unpleasant everyday situations by fantasizing that she was another person. She also had "bad nerves," feeling very tense a great deal of the time, and she felt inferior and lacked self-confidence. Evelyn's parents were divorced when she was two, and her mother had one, and her father two, subsequent remarriages and divorces. She felt that her parents both tried to exact gratitude from her for the material things they gave her in place of love, and she was physically afraid of her father. She planned to be married after her graduation. She was diagnosed as an anxiety neurosis, was accepted for the study and assigned to a psychotherapist.

Caroline Gray was excluded from the study because of her vagueness in describing her problems and because these problems stemmed primarily from a temporary situation. Although she and her husband were being divorced, he continued to call her, visit her, have sexual relations with her, and abuse her verbally and blame her for his sexual inadequacies. She continually felt that he used and took advantage of her. This feeling was certainly justified, and she seemed to have no other symptoms and was therefore not accepted for the study. Her assessor urged that she refuse to see her husband for a month. Having accomplished this, she called the assessor again and eventually had an extremely helpful course of brief psychotherapy with him.

### *Demographic Characteristics*

The patients in the sample were predominantly in their early 20's, female (60%), and white. Only seven blacks were included in the final sample, all of them female. This black-white ratio reflected that of the clinic. Although Temple is situated in a predominantly black, lower-class area, its Community Mental Health Center handles the psychotherapy of most of its local catchment area. Only patients considered especially difficult or atypical in some way are referred to the outpatient clinic. The clinic itself serves a citywide referral area.

Most patients (71%) were born and raised in a large city, with some (23%) from small cities and a few (6%) from small towns or rural areas. A majority (52%) were living at home with their family of origin at the time of initial assessment. Family of origin included on the average two siblings. Only 26% had been married at the time of initial assessment; of these, 22% had separated from their marital partners and were living alone. Over half (57%) of the married patients had at least one child.

Most of the patients professed some religious belief. The most frequent association was with the Jewish faith (47%); Protestants and Roman Catholics were equally represented (17% and 16%, respectively), and 21% of the patients expressed no formal religious affiliation. Patients had completed an average of 14 years of education, that is, about two years of college or other post-secondary school training. Estimates of intellectual ability as assessed by the Mill Hill Vocabulary Scale suggested a mean verbal IQ of approximately 99. This figure appears somewhat low, considering the educational achievement of these patients. IQ estimates from this test probably tend to underestimate the intellectual level of American samples; there is some suggestion that the test's norms, established on a British population, are higher than norms for American samples.

There were 27% of the patients working full-time. Roughly one third (37%) were economically self-supporting, another third (32%) were completely dependent upon others for their support, and the middle third were partially self-supporting. The majority of patients in the latter groups were students, who made up 54% of the total sample. It proved difficult to obtain an accurate index of the income or occupational level of the sample. In the case of students or young people who were not yet completely self-supporting, the income range and occupational status of the head of the family of origin was used. However, many of these young people were unaware of the salary level of the head of the family or even of what his precise occupational category was. In many cases they were unable even to estimate their fathers' income ranges. The sample's average income range ($5,000 to $6,000 per annum) is based both upon patients who were completely self-supporting, and upon the head of household as estimated by those who were not self-supporting, and is probably not an accurate estimate.

## DIAGNOSIS

### *Minnesota Multiphasic Personality Inventory*

The MMPI was used in judging psychological characteristics. Means and standard deviations of the nine clinical MMPI scales for each of the three treatment groups and the overall sample are shown in Table 1. The overall means show considerable pathology in the patient group. Four of the nine subscale mean scores (depression, psychopathic deviate, psychasthenia, and schizophrenia) are within the abnormal range, i.e., more than two standard deviations above the test mean of 50. The mean score for all pathology scales (excluding the masculinity-femininity scale) is 70.09, indicating that the overall pathology level was quite high. Two-thirds of the patients scored abnormally high on the depression scale, while well over half scored abnormally high on the psychopathic deviate, psychasthenia, and schizophrenia scales. Only 8 of the

TABLE 1. MMPI Clinical Scale Scores of Patients at Initial Assessment

| | Behavior Therapy | | Psycho-therapy | | Wait List | | Overall | |
|---|---|---|---|---|---|---|---|---|
| | $\bar{X}$ | $s$ | $\bar{X}$ | $s$ | $\bar{X}$ | $s$ | $\bar{X}$ | $s$ |
| Hypochondriasis | 60.14 | 12.55 | 60.89 | 13.40 | 61.46 | 11.10 | 60.83 | 12.52 |
| Depression | 76.93 | 15.02 | 79.19 | 11.97 | 82.50 | 15.95 | 79.54 | 14.53 |
| Hysteria | 65.50 | 10.34 | 68.22 | 12.41 | 65.18 | 7.76 | 66.30 | 10.41 |
| Psychopathic Deviate | 75.11 | 12.08 | 76.52 | 12.97 | 74.79 | 14.88 | 75.47 | 13.38 |
| Masculinity-Femininity | 58.32 | 17.67 | 56.22 | 19.38 | 54.07 | 18.61 | 56.20 | 18.64 |
| Paranoia | 62.82 | 9.96 | 63.89 | 10.87 | 67.14 | 9.82 | 64.62 | 10.38 |
| Psychasthenia | 75.32 | 11.94 | 74.96 | 12.99 | 77.32 | 14.72 | 75.87 | 13.32 |
| Schizophrenia | 77.79 | 15.43 | 76.48 | 17.93 | 78.11 | 16.91 | 77.46 | 16.77 |
| Mania | 59.07 | 11.80 | 64.48 | 11.30 | 58.50 | 12.38 | 60.68 | 11.88 |

Note: In this and following tables $\bar{X}$ represents the mean, $s$ the standard deviation, *df* degrees of freedom, *M.S.* mean square from analysis of variance, and $F$ the $F$ ratio also from analysis of variance.

90 patients scored within the normal range on all clinical scales. The mean score on the social introversion scale of the MMPI (Table 2) is approximately one and one-half standard deviations above the mean.

### *Eysenck Personality Inventory*

Group means and standard deviations of patients' scores on several personality tests are shown in Table 2. In its first two rows, results of the extraversion and neuroticism scores of the Eysenck Personality Inventory are presented in percentile form in terms of norms for American college students. Patients score below average on the extraversion scale, supporting the evidence from the MMPI social introversion scale that they are more introverted than the average college student. Neuroticism scores indicate considerable degree of pathology in all three patient groups: the overall mean score is at the eighty-sixth percentile.

### *California Psychological Inventory*

Scores on the scales of the California Psychological Inventory suggest that the sample shows low self-control, sociability, and socialization (Table 2). These characteristics seem compatible with the description of the patients provided by other measures. However, the self-acceptance scale, which might be expected to be low in a group seeking psychiatric help, is close to the normal average.

### *Psychiatric Diagnosis*

The assessors diagnosed each patient according to American Psychiatric Association standards (DSMII). By this criterion the sample consisted of approximately two-thirds neurotics and one-third personality disorders.

TABLE 2. Psychometric Scores of Patient Groups at Initial Assessment

| | Behavior Therapy | | Psycho-therapy | | Wait List | | Overall | |
|---|---|---|---|---|---|---|---|---|
| | $\bar{X}$ | $s$ | $\bar{X}$ | $s$ | $\bar{X}$ | $s$ | $\bar{X}$ | $s$ |
| *Eysenck Personality Inventory* | | | | | | | | |
| Extraversion | 35.13 | 27.17 | 46.48 | 32.07 | 36.83 | 26.00 | 39.48 | 28.96 |
| Neuroticism | 85.37 | 17.83 | 84.52 | 17.43 | 87.93 | 17.80 | 85.94 | 18.29 |
| *Minnesota Multiphasic Personality Inventory* | | | | | | | | |
| Social Introversion | 64.21 | 12.46 | 63.59 | 11.04 | 66.50 | 9.83 | 64.77 | 11.24 |
| Manifest Anxiety | 27.79 | 9.58 | 30.11 | 8.09 | 31.04 | 7.39 | 29.64 | 8.53 |
| *California Psychological Inventory* | | | | | | | | |
| Self-acceptance | 46.18 | 12.84 | 51.37 | 9.78 | 47.30 | 10.83 | 48.28 | 11.49 |
| Self-control | 38.79 | 11.26 | 36.19 | 10.54 | 37.33 | 10.45 | 37.44 | 10.73 |
| Socialization | 40.68 | 12.72 | 42.26 | 12.15 | 37.52 | 11.77 | 40.15 | 12.52 |
| Sociability | 37.11 | 10.61 | 32.96 | 10.68 | 33.15 | 11.82 | 34.41 | 11.28 |

| *Diagnosis* | *Number of patients* |
|---|---|
| Anxiety reaction | 57 |
| Depressive neurosis | 4 |
| Phobic neurosis | 2 |
| Depersonalization neurosis | 1 |
| Hysterical personality | 8 |
| Obsessive-compulsive personality | 5 |
| Schizoid personality | 1 |
| Passive-aggressive personality (also passive-dependent) | 7 |
| Inadequate personality | 1 |
| Cyclothymic personality | 1 |
| Paranoid personality | 1 |
| Immature personality | 1 |
| Adjustment reaction | 2 |
| Marital maladjustment | 1 |
| Special symptom reactions (obesity, impotence) | 2 |
| Total neuroses | 64 |
| Total personality disorders | 25 |
| Total miscellaneous diagnoses | 5 |
| TOTAL | 94 |

## TYPE OF TARGET SYMPTOMS

Type of target symptom is another index for classifying patients' problems, and an informal tabulation of symptoms gives a feeling for the general nature of the sample. In order of decreasing frequency, these patients reported as important symptoms: generalized anxiety, interpersonal difficulties with everyone, low self-esteem, interpersonal difficulties with opposite-sex peers, depression and sadness, somatic complaints, difficulties with family of origin, poor school or work performance, anxiety about nonsocial situations (animal phobias, subways, sneezing), difficulties with spouse and children, homosexual concern, indecisiveness, problems with goals or career choice, difficulties with sexual performance, and obesity. There were other target symptoms that could not be placed in these categories, but none was present in more than two patients.

In a more formal attempt to summarize the nature of the three target symptoms the patient selected at initial assessment and in the hope of discovering whether either therapy is particularly successful in any one area, these symptoms were classified according to three major categories: the context in which the symptom appeared, the kind of symptom, and the mode of action of the symptom. Each symptom was classified according to each of the three categories.

Table 3 shows the target symptoms in context. The "context" refers to the area of life in which the symptom was present, and includes the following subcategories:

1. School. Problems directly related to performance in the academic environment (fear of exams, poor school performance).

TABLE 3. Number of Target Symptoms in Each Context

| Context | Behavior Therapy | Psycho-therapy | Wait List | Overall | Percent |
|---|---|---|---|---|---|
| School | 5 | 11 | 4 | 20 | 7.4 |
| Work | 2 | 4 | 1 | 7 | 2.6 |
| Family of origin | 9 | 5 | 2 | 16 | 5.9 |
| Peers | 10 | 6 | 14 | 30 | 11.1 |
| Married family | 7 | 6 | 2 | 15 | 5.6 |
| Sex | 10 | 4 | 8 | 22 | 8.1 |
| Other people | 8 | 18 | 13 | 31 | 11.5 |
| Self | 13 | 9 | 11 | 33 | 12.2 |
| Other specific context | 6 | 5 | 10 | 21 | 7.8 |
| Not applicable | 20 | 22 | 25 | 67 | 24.8 |

2. Work. Difficulties in work adjustment (criticism by fellow teachers, "not conscientious enough at my work").

3. Family of origin. Problems associated with the relations between the patient and his parents or siblings ("frequent fights when I talk to my mother," "I rely on my mother to make decisions").

4. Peers. Problems associated with the patient's relationships with people of his own age group. Problems relating to the opposite sex are included, but problems specifically related to sexual performance are excluded (lack of close friends, loneliness).

5. Married Family. Problems in relations with spouse and children (feeling guilty toward children about divorce, fear of killing children).

6. Sex. (Conflicts over homosexuality, impotence).

7. Other people. Symptoms not specifically related to peers or family ("I get angry at people," "I'm uncomfortable with groups where I might be called upon to speak").

8. Self. Symptoms which refer to dissatisfaction with the self in some specific context. ("Overweight and can't stay on a diet," "I don't have the ability to make decisions").

9. Other specific context. Problems that occur in a specific context but do not fit in other categories (difficulty in falling asleep, fear of traveling in the subway).

10. Not applicable. This category refers to symptoms which do not occur in a specific context. ("I feel tense and jittery all the time," "I feel life is hopeless").

*The kind of symptom* fell into ten general classifications, as shown in Table 4.

1. Anxiety. Problems reflecting generalized tension or anxiety as well as those refering to specific fears. ("I'm extremely tense in crowded rooms," "I'm very nervous").

2. Depression. Symptoms that might be interpreted as in-

TABLE 4. Number of Each Kind of Target Symptom

| Symptom | Behavior Therapy | Psycho-therapy | Wait List | Overall | Percent |
|---|---|---|---|---|---|
| Anxiety | 18 | 13 | 24 | 55 | 20.4 |
| Depression | 3 | 4 | 4 | 11 | 4.1 |
| Anger | 7 | 9 | 5 | 21 | 7.8 |
| Bodily complaints | 10 | 10 | 9 | 29 | 10.7 |
| Unwanted acts | 6 | 8 | 19 | 33 | 12.2 |
| Worries | 13 | 8 | 3 | 24 | 8.9 |
| Lack of behavior | 18 | 17 | 10 | 45 | 16.7 |
| Indecision | 4 | 3 | 5 | 12 | 4.4 |
| Self-confidence | 7 | 12 | 5 | 24 | 8.9 |
| Other | 4 | 6 | 6 | 16 | 5.9 |

dicating a state of depression. ("I feel unhappy, depressed and miserable," "I'm tired and listless").

3. Anger. Expressions of hostility, aggression, and anger. ("I argue with everyone, particularly with my mother and sister," "I can't control my temper").

4. Bodily complaints. Specific dissatisfaction with some function of the body, such as ulcer or palpitations.

5. Unwanted acts. Habits or specific behavior of the patient that he would like to get rid of. ("I drink too much," "I pull out my hair").

6. Worries. Excessive rumination about events or unwanted thoughts, ("I worry about something happening to my wife and child," "I worry over sexual relationship with my husband").

7. Lack of behavior. Inability to perform satisfactorily in a given area of behavior. ("I just sit and can't work," "I can't form close friendships").

8. Indecision. Difficulty in making up one's mind. ("I always doubt myself before taking action," "I rely on my mother to make decisions").

9. Self-confidence problem. Feelings of inferiority, lack of confidence in social situations.

10. Other dissatisfactions. Problems that do not readily fit into the other nine categories.

Table 5 shows the modes of action of the presenting difficulties. The subcategories are as follows:

1. Cognition. Worries, and other thoughts of the patient.
2. Emotion. Expressions of fear, irritability, and other feelings.
3. Behavior. Symptoms reflected in overt action on the part of the patient.
4. Physiological reaction. Difficulties with bodily functioning.

*Distribution of Target Symptoms*

In terms of context, problems concerned with the self, mainly questions of self-confidence and decision-making ability, are most frequent, as shown in Table 3. Problems with other people in general and with peers are the next most frequent areas. The majority of problems, in fact, have to do with some form of interpersonal difficulties. Table 4 presents the frequency with which different kinds of problems are treated by each of the three treatment groups. The most frequent pro-

TABLE 5. Number of Target Symptoms in Each Area of Functioning

| Area | Behavior Therapy | Psycho-therapy | Wait List | Overall | Percent |
|---|---|---|---|---|---|
| Cognition | 12 | 10 | 7 | 29 | 10.7 |
| Emotion | 39 | 44 | 42 | 125 | 46.3 |
| Behavior | 30 | 29 | 33 | 92 | 34.1 |
| Physiological reaction | 9 | 7 | 8 | 24 | 8.9 |

blem involves some form of anxiety, including both generalized anxiety and fears of specific objects or situations.

The areas in which the presenting difficulties occur are presented in Table 5. Nearly half these problems involve some form of emotion or affective disturbance; roughly one-third involved some disorder of overt behavior. Physiological reactions and cognitive disturbances are both less frequent.

We were surprised at how long our patients had had their symptoms. Only four patients said that all their difficulties had been present for less than a year. On the other hand, sixty-three claimed that all their difficulties had been present for longer than one year. The remaining patients presented a combination of difficulties of both relatively recent onset and a long-standing nature. These patients illustrated well the long-standing complaints of those who come to psychotherapy.

Table 6 shows the mean severity of the first target symptom, and of all three target symptoms, as rated by the assessor at the initial interview. It can be seen that the average patient's tar-

TABLE 6. Severity of Target Symptoms: Initial Assessor Ratings

| | | Behavior Therapy | Psycho-therapy | Wait List |
|---|---|---|---|---|
| First symptom | $\bar{X}$ | 3.10 | 3.17 | 3.13 |
| | $s$ | .48 | .65 | .86 |
| Three symptoms | $\bar{X}$ | 8.81 | 9.13 | 8.82 |
| | $s$ | 1.39 | 1.65 | 2.01 |

Severity rating
0 = absent
1 = doubtful or trivial
2 = mild
3 = moderate
4 = severe

get symptoms were all rated between "moderately severe" and "severe" at initial assessment.

### *Previous Treatment*

Sixty-four percent of the patients said they had previously taken part in formal psychotherapy. Of these, 41% had been in treatment for ten hours or less, while 59% had had more extensive treatment.

Of the patients who had not received treatment, 9% had visited a psychiatrist on at least one occasion. Thus, participation in the study represented the first contact with psychiatry for only 27% of the patients. Eight percent of these had sought out sources of informal treatment in the community with clergymen, friends, or relatives. Unexpectedly, only 7% of patients with previous psychiatric contact had received medication. This seems a remarkably low figure in view of the widespread use of psychoactive agents in psychiatry.

## INITIAL ASSESSMENT

On the morning of the appointment the research assistant met the patient and his friend or relative about half an hour before the time of the appointment with the assessor. She took the patient's family and general medical history and collected demographic information such as his religion, occupation, and income. The patient and relative were then assigned to separate rooms and given the Eysenck Personality Inventory. When this was completed the research assistant talked informally to the patient for a short time and tried to prepare him for the interview with the psychiatrist. If patients were apprehensive she tried to calm them, speaking in a friendly and informal way. She explained that there would be a tape recorder present to make an accurate record, but that the recording would be completely confidential. She did not discuss their problems, except those directly concerned with the procedures involved in the psychiatric assessment. She answered any questions as directly as possible, in order to help the patient to understand what was happening, and to feel as comfortable as possible. She also explained that there was a great demand for doctors and that sometimes there was a waiting list. She added that it might not be possible to get treatment at once, but that all patients who were accepted for treatment would be given treatment.

The research assistant then introduced the patient to the assessing psychiatrist. The assessor at first conducted an open-ended interview, inviting the patient to talk freely about the problems for which he was seeking help. The patient was encouraged to give a sketch of his background and describe the members of his family, how they got on with each other, and his own place in the family. After this general discussion, the assessor and patient together decided on the three target symptoms. The assessor then rated their severity and administered the SSIAM. Several other measures were taken at this interview.

Anxiety in some form was usually expressed by the patient. If tension, nervousness, or anxiety was not listed as one of the three target complaints, the assessor specifically inquired about it and made the same type of ratings used for each target symptom.

Feeling at ease came next. The patient was asked, "When did you last feel completely at ease?" and "For how long do you feel completely at ease nowadays?" These times were then rated.

Previous treatment was another object of inquiry. The patient was asked to describe the kind and extent of any psychotherapy he had previously received, including informal treatment from a doctor or clergyman.

The assessor then presented a checklist of autonomic and related symptoms divided into two parts, one to be completed by the patient, the other by the assessor. The patient's part had 106 questions ("Do you get uncomfortable or tight feelings in your chest?" "Is it difficult to relax?" "Do you toss and turn in bed at night?") which the patient answered rapidly by checking either "yes" or "no." The psychiatrist made some 50 more ratings on the second part of the checklist. Some of these items required direct observation: pulse rate, sweaty palms, tremor of extended hands. This list included symptoms which are more easily rated by a psychiatrist after discussion with the patient than by the patient alone, for example, the hyperventilation syndrome, obsessions, compulsions, sexual symptoms, dissatisfaction with some part of the body.

Several of the above measures were included to obtain data for a separate study of symptom patterns in neurosis.

At this assessment the patient was also given the MMPI, the CPI, and the Mill-Hill Vocabulary Scale. (Again for purposes incidental to this study a 602-item "inquiry" was given, concerned with everyday occurrences which might disturb the patient.)

After this interview the assessor made a formal diagnosis in terms of the American Psychiatric Association's *Diagnostic and Statistical Manual, 2nd ed.,* and wrote a case history and anamnestic description of the patient.

If a patient was found suitable for the study according to the criteria described earlier, the assessor immediately informed him that he would be offered therapy. He was also told that since therapists only became available as other patients finished therapy, his name might be put on a waiting list to be given therapy as soon as possible, and certainly within four months. The assessor added that there was a good chance that a therapist would be available almost immediately, but that if the patient had to wait, the research assistant would keep in touch with him by telephone, and he should feel free to call the assessor or the 24-hour-a-day Crisis Center in case of an emergency or crisis. This concluded the patient's initial assessment.

*Informant Interview*

While the patient and assessor were talking, in another room the research assistant was interviewing a close friend or relative (in most cases a parent, spouse, or roommate) of the patient. They first talked about how long (average 12 years) and intimately the informant and patient had known one another, and then informally discussed the patient's life, his adjustment, and his problems as seen by the informant. The research assistant administered the SSIAM, which the informant answered as it applied to the patient. He also answered the 106-question checklist as if from the patient's point of view.

This interview was intended to provide another vantage point from which to view each patient, and also to show whether or not information obtained from people in this relation to a patient would differ (e.g., be more or less optimistic) from data collected from other raters—from the therapist, independent assessor, or the patient himself.

## ASSIGNMENT TO TREATMENT

While the assessor and the patient were concluding the first interview, the research assistant was assigning the patient to treatment. She either explained the wait list procedure to him or gave him the name and telephone number of the therapist who would be expecting his call.

Patients were randomly assigned to treatment groups. It would have been desirable to equalize the groups, not only as to number of patients, but with respect to each of the variables which might influence therapeutic outcome. Age, sex, education, symptoms, personality type, severity of illness—the list of possibly relevant features is endless. To equalize all these factors among treatment groups would require an infinitely large patient sample. The problem was complicated by the necessity of assigning patients to treatment as they were accepted into the study, rather than holding them in abeyance until the entire sample had been collected (nineteen months) and until sample distributions could be determined for the various measures.

We decided to match treatment groups only in respect to number of patients, sex, and severity of neurosis, hoping that otherwise random assignment would equally distribute other characteristics among the three treatment groups.

The neuroticism scale of the Eysenck Personality Inventory was the standard by which groups were matched for severity of pathology. This scale has the advantage of being simple to administer and score, thus providing a quick measure of severity. A *z* score of 92 on the neuroticism scale was selected as the cut-off point to differentiate between high- and low-pathology patients. (This was the median score in an earlier study using a similar sample of patients.)[2]

We set up the study in nine subgroups: three for the psychotherapists, three for the behavior therapists, and three (entirely arbitrary) subgroups of the wait list. Of the ten patients in each subgroup, five would be male and five female, five would have neuroticism *z* scores over 92, and five would have scores under 92. However, as the study proceeded it became obvious that, reflecting the national figures for outpatient psychiatric treatment, there were more female patients available than male patients. The assignment procedure was modified to take this into account, allowing six females and four male patients in each of the nine subgroups. In the final assignment each of the six therapists and each of the three wait-list subgroups received three female patients with high pathology, three female patients with low pathology, two male patients with high pathology, and two male patients with low pathology. The design is illustrated in Table 7. The method of random assignment to groups is described in Appendix 2.

An additional four patients who were available at the close of the selection phase were also admitted to the study. Three of these patients were assigned to the wait list and one to the behavior therapy group, as insurance against early dropouts. However, the anticipated loss of patients did not occur at four months and since the design for the main factorial analysis at four months was set up for ninety patients, these additional patients were not included in that analysis.

Tables 1 and 2 illustrate the success of this random assignment method in equalizing the treatment groups for certain factors which might influence therapeutic outcome. The largest difference between any two groups on any of the MMPI scales is less than 6 points, with a standard deviation of over 15. There was a slight tendency for patients assigned to the psychotherapy group to be more extraverted (as measured on the Eysenck extraversion scale) than the behavior therapy patients, but this tendency was far from significant ($t = 1.4790, p > .10$). Because of the method used to assign patients to groups, the three groups naturally have very similar scores on the Eysenck neuroticism scale. The groups' means are very similar on all four scales of the California Psychological Inventory.

Table 6 shows the mean severity for each treatment group of the first target symptom and of all three target symptoms, as rated by the assessor at the initial interview. Average target symptom severity was similar for patients in the three groups.

TABLE 7. Number of Patients in Each Treatment Subgroup

| Therapist Experience | Pathology | Behavior Therapy | | Psycho-therapy | | Wait List | |
|---|---|---|---|---|---|---|---|
| | | M[a] | F[b] | M | F | M | F |
| High | High | 2 | 3 | 2 | 3 | 2 | 3 |
| | Low | 2 | 3 | 2 | 3 | 2 | 3 |
| Intermediate | High | 2 | 3 | 2 | 3 | 2 | 3 |
| | Low | 2 | 3 | 2 | 3 | 2 | 3 |
| Low | High | 2 | 3 | 2 | 3 | 2 | 3 |
| | Low | 2 | 3 | 2 | 3 | 2 | 3 |

[a]male
[b]female

There were no marked differences in extent of psychiatric experience among the three groups of patients. The following patients are illustrative.

Marie Sutton was a striking, dark-haired, 24-year-old opera singer enrolled at a major music school. She complained of a frequent feeling that she was about to pass out, especially while performing on stage. This feeling, a sensation like being hit on the head, followed by nausea, occurred several times a day and lasted several minutes. She never actually did faint, but this feeling plus her ever-present extreme general tension, interfered with practicing and performing and made her whole life uncomfortable. She had difficulty concentrating and usually was able to practice for only 10 minutes at a time. The only time she was ever completely at ease was when she was with her boyfriend.

Marie was given up for adoption at birth. Her foster father was rather passive and dominated by his wife, but sometimes took Marie's side against her foster mother who was cold and strict, and who beat her. The hated foster mother died when Marie was 14, and she had weekly psychotherapy from 15 to 17 without much success. She kept house for her foster father, but they had a rather distant relationship, and she was not entirely happy with her boyfriend of eight years. Marie was diagnosed as an anxiety neurosis and was assigned to psychotherapy.

Emma Hubbard was an extremely fat college freshman living at home with her parents. Her obesity (225 pounds at assessment) was her main problem. Her other target symptoms were self-consciousness about her appearance and complete lack of male companionship. Emma had been overweight even as a baby, and everyone else in her family was fat. Her father had been sick and unable to work the last eight years, and Emma had helped her domineering mother in the family's delicatessen, eating all the while. Her assessor made the diagnosis of special symptom reaction: obesity. He predicted that she would not lose weight in short-term therapy. Emma was assigned to the wait list.

Tom Morton was 20 and lived with his parents at the time of his first assessment. He was a tall, hypercasual college senior with a neat beard. He had an impressive academic record and had already been accepted by several medical schools. He suffered from strong feelings of loneliness, of not knowing what his values were, of the need to impress everyone that he was "tops." He had once been briefly hospitalized for a "hyperactive state," and showed some signs of inappropriate elation during his assessment. Tom was struggling for complete independence from his parents. He felt much closer to his mother than to his father, whom he described as unhappy, frustrated, and rather like a dictator. Tom was diagnosed as a probable cyclothymic personality and was assigned to behavior therapy.

Raymond Simpson, a weak-looking 20-year-old college student with severe acne, had a rather typical anxiety neurosis. When he was with people he felt nervous, his eyes twitched, and he blinked frequently. He was often depressed and felt himself a failure, inferior to other people. He described both parents as domineering ("talking to them is like talking to a brick wall") and when at home he "locked himself up in a shell" and refused to associate with them. His mother had often been hospitalized for nervous breakdowns and colitis, and his father suffered from monthly migraines with great tension. On the positive side, Raymond had a good emotional and sexual relationship with his girlfriend and they were tentatively engaged. Raymond was assigned to a psychotherapist.

Veneta Williams was a 45-year-old unmarried black social

worker suffering from depression, jitteriness, suspiciousness, uncertainty about her career, and feelings of inadequacy at work. Seven years before, she had attempted suicide by stabbing herself in the chest with a carving knife, and spent several weeks in the hospital. She never repeated the attempt, however, and was not suicidal at the time of assessment. She complained with some bitterness that she took care of various members of her large family but they did not take care of her. In the past several years she had had a series of operations, a hysterectomy, breast biopsies, and two mastectomies. The assessor felt that these had contributed to her depression. Miss Williams's brother described the same general problems to the research assistant, adding that she changed jobs and friends too often, and seemed to have little interest in male companionship. Miss Williams was diagnosed a reactive depression and was assigned to psychotherapy.

Norman Rollins, 31, was a slight, tense, pinched-looking government clerk, who also attended college at night. He was happily married and loved his child. He suffered overwhelming anxiety in nearly every social situation: saying hello to a friend, making small talk, sitting in a room with other people, or talking to anyone except when giving a specialized opinion. He also worried terribly about something harmful happening to his wife or child. He was often upset by thinking about having to do things that were expected of him, from sexual intercourse to going to the supermarket. Such requirements made him uncomfortable, weak and defensive, and led to long unproductive arguments with his wife. In her interview with the research assistant, Mrs. Rollins painted the same picture as her husband had, adding that he was self-centered and that she felt less relaxed with him than with other people. Mr. Rollins had an unstable background. He was an illegitimate child and never knew his father, and his mother's subsequent marriage broke up when Norman was 8. He was in foster homes between the ages of 13 and 17, and then spent five years in the navy. He was diagnosed as an anxiety neurosis and assigned to psychotherapy.

Louise Shaw, 33, was a dark, rather dumpy housewife with two children, who suffered from a variety of fears. For three years she had been afraid to go out because she might lose control of her urine. (She had actually had two incidents of incontinence, following the births of her children, but the fear did not begin until much later.) She was afraid to be in crowds, afraid to speak out because of possible criticism, and had recently begun to fear death. Her marriage, by comparison, seemed happy. Mr. Shaw, a patient, easygoing man, gave the research assistant the same general description of his wife's problems. Mrs. Shaw's parents were divorced when she was 15. She rarely saw her father after this, but had a warm, close relationship with her mother. Mrs. Shaw's diagnosis was anxiety, phobic neurosis, and she was assigned to behavior therapy.

Mary Teresa Moore was a beautiful girl of 19, but with a worried, nervous look. She had been depressed and anxious for about three months, had lost 15 pounds, and had trouble sleeping. She found it hard to fall asleep and waked at 5:00 in the morning. She planned to be married in a few months, but although her fiancé was a good Catholic, her twin sister, a nun, was urging her to put off the marriage. She felt guilty about feeling sexual desire, despite her lack of sexual experience. She had had obsessive thoughts about cutting off her fingers, or her future children's fingers, and of shutting her children into small spaces where they would suffocate. She felt depersonalized, as if she weren't really herself, felt as if her head were charged, felt as if God wanted her to go out of her mind, and then felt guilty for all these feelings. Prayer made her feel worse. She had had a happy home life, had done well in high school, had had lots of friends and dates. Mary Teresa was diagnosed as a mixed psychoneurosis with anxiety, depression, and obsessional and phobic thoughts, and she was assigned to psychotherapy.

## THERAPISTS

All the therapists in the study were white males, and all but one were psychiatrists. In addition to their formal credentials, all were considered good therapists by their peers, and all enjoyed excellent professional reputations. The senior behavior therapist was widely experienced, and at the time of the study he had treated an estimated 2,000 neurotic patients over the course of 20 years' practice of behavior therapy. The second behavior therapist was the only psychologist (PhD) among the six. In recent years some of his therapeutic strategies included cognitive restructuring, but his therapy was still strongly behavioral in style and method. He had treated about 1,000 patients during 13 years. The third had treated about 250 patients in his six years of behavior therapy practice. While he occasionally used cognitive restructuring, his overall technique was classically behavioral.

The senior psychoanalytically oriented therapist was a member of the American Psychoanalytic Association. He had treated some 6,000 patients over his 35 years of practice, some in classical psychoanalysis and many in psychoanalytically oriented psychotherapy. The second psychotherapist had trained abroad and was a member of the International Psychoanalytic Association. He had treated approximately 500 patients in 20 years, many by classical analysis, and, in recent years, more by analytically oriented therapeutic methods. The junior psychotherapist was undergoing personal analysis with a training analyst. He had treated some 300 patients in his eight years of practice, mostly by psychoanalytically oriented psychotherapy. Each therapist took the Eysenck Personality Inventory and the A-B Scale of the Strong Vocational Interest Blank. Since only the two least experienced therapists were B's and the other four were all A's in Whitehorn and Betz's terms, the A-B variable was confounded with therapist experience, and could not be examined independently. All therapists scored rather low on extraversion and very low on neuroticism on the Eysenck, with scores clustered so closely together that the relation of these variables to patients' outcome could not be studied.

### *The Therapies*

In the ideal study the therapists within each treatment group would be restricted to the use of a single technique, so that any group differences in outcome could be attributed to the use of these techniques. For example, if behavior therapists used only systematic desensitization with all patients, the results could be evaluated in terms of the efficacy of systematic desensitization relative to analytically oriented short-term therapy. As is so often the case in clinical research, the ideal study was virtually impossible. Therapists were understandably reluctant to treat all patients with a technique which would not be optimally useful for each. To provide a sufficiently large sample of patients for whom a single technique, say systematic desensitization, would be the most appropriate procedure would have required many more years of beating the outpatient bushes. In addition, one of the major aims of the study was to evaluate the two therapies using a sample of mixed neurotic patients who typically receive a "talking therapy" in outpatient clinics rather than a restricted sample with unusual characteristics.

Consequently, therapists were free to use whatever therapeutic techniques they felt to be most appropriate for each individual patient. This allowed them the freedom to treat patients to the best of their ability with no artificial restrictions upon their usual clinical skills. Freedom is not without its drawbacks, since we were now faced with the problem of determining just what happened in therapy, and insuring that distinctive treatments were given by each group of therapists. In terms of "who can do what, and with which, unto whom" we must specify the "which" as precisely as possible.

To insure that there was no misunderstanding among therapists as to what constituted behavior therapy and what belonged to analytically oriented therapy, a list of stipulative definitions of each treatment was drawn up. An oversimple summary could be put as follows, naming only some of the principal points of divergence.

| *Behavior Therapy* | *Psychotherapy* |
|---|---|
| Specific advice | Advice infrequent |
| Resistance not interpreted | Resistance interpretation used |
| Dream interpretation not used | Encourage report of dreams, which may or may not be used |
| Relaxation specifically taught | Relaxation not a direct aim |
| Desensitization directly undertaken | Desensitization indirect through congeniality of interview with therapist |
| Practical retraining undertaken | Retraining not emphasized |
| Encourage report of symptoms, to be explained biologically | Symptoms if reported at all may be interpreted symbolically |
| No emphasis on childhood memories | Memories of interest; further ones are sought |
| Deliberate attempt to curb behavior that results in anxiety | Behavior control rarely tried |
| Assertive training undertaken | Only indirect encouragement of assertive action in everyday life |

A more complete list, reproduced in Appendix 3, defines what procedures and techniques are common to both therapies, and those allowable only within one or the other. Therapists approved these descriptions and felt they would not be restricted in their treatment.

In order to provide an independent measure of in-therapy behavior, tape recordings were made of the fifth interview between patient and therapist. These were transcribed and rated on a number of dimensions: the Truax variables (depth of interpersonal contact, accurate empathy, unconditional positive regard, and therapist self-congruence), nonlexical speech characteristics, the Lennard and Bernstein Scale of Therapist Informational Specificity, and a modified Bales interaction scale (the "Temple Content Categories"). Therapists also rated their attitudes toward their patients, while patients completed the Truax Relationship Questionnaire and the Lorr Scale, both designed to measure patient perception of therapist behavior. The purpose of these measures, to be described in detail later, was to test for differences between behavior therapists and psychotherapists in their pattern of interaction with patients.

Following completion of four months' therapy with each patient, therapists were interviewed by the assessor who had followed that patient. He obtained information about the therapist's conception of the patient's problem, his general therapeutic strategy, and specific techniques used.

## THE WAIT LIST

The wait list might more accurately be called a "minimal contact" group than a "no treatment" group. When they were assigned to the wait list, these patients had already had a long interview with the assessor and had been promised treatment. When they were told they would have to wait four months because of the shortage of doctors, it was emphasized that they would definitely receive treatment at the end of that period, and that if any crisis occurred they were free to call their assessors or the department's emergency unit for help. During the waiting period, they were called every few weeks by the research assistant, a warm friendly person whom they had talked with before the assessment interview. She asked them how they were getting along, and reminded them that they were not forgotten and would soon be assigned to treatment. These contacts were made out of responsibility to these patients whose treatment was postponed for research reasons, and also to insure that all control patients in fact would wait four months to be assigned to treatment rather than give up. Here the patients were involved in a personal and committed, though brief, relationship that undoubtedly contributed to the 100 percent continuity.

Both the assessor and the research assistant avoided any explicit therapy, such as advice or interpretations, with the control patients. Nevertheless some of the patients felt these contacts had been therapeutic, and it is true that most of the nonspecific aspects of therapy were present, although for short periods. The assessment was in many ways the equivalent of a first therapy interview, with its novel experience of unburdening oneself to an uninvolved but sympathetic listener, sorting out one's problems, and the insights that sometimes come unbidden in such an environment. In addition, these patients experienced arousal of hope, expectation of help, the feeling that there was someone to call on in the event of a crisis—the usual concomitants of beginning therapy. Also they could count on a regular, though short, conversation with an interested person.

## LENGTH OF TREATMENT

Behavior therapy and psychotherapy patients were given four months of weekly, hour-long therapy (an average of 13.2 and 14.2 sessions, respectively), and control patients spent four months on the wait list. We intended to exclude as dropouts only those patients who attended fewer than four sessions, and no patients were in fact excluded as dropouts. We purposely set this criterion low in order to exclude only those patients who were not serious about therapy or who were frightened away before therapy had a chance really to begin. To set a higher standard for inclusion might give one treatment an unfair advantage by eliminating from consideration, as dropouts, a large proportion of those for whom therapy was not going well and who would have shown up as "failures" had they completed the course of therapy rather than giving up sooner.

## FOUR-MONTH REASSESSMENT

Four months after the initial assessment the patient saw his original assessor again. He was not formally prohibited from discussing his treatment, but the assessor tried to avoid such discussion and to remain blind wherever possible, with surprising success. Before the interview the assessor usually reread the history and description he had written about the patient after the initial assessment, but he did not have access to his original numerical ratings on any of the scales.

Again the assessment began with an unstructured conversation about changes in the last four months and how the patient was doing now. Then the assessor rated the target symptoms, as before, on an absolute severity scale. In addition, he and the patient each rated each of the target symptoms on a thirteen-point comparative scale of severity ranging from "completely recovered" to "very much worse" than at the initial assessment. They also both rated work, social, sexual, and overall adjustment on thirteen-point comparative scales.

The SSIAM was administered again, as were the scales for anxiety and feeling at ease, and the checklist of emotional symptoms. The patient was also asked which, if any, of a list of twenty-five potentially disturbing events had occurred in his life in the past four months. These included, for example, engagement, divorce, major illness, moving, first job, and death in family. After the interview, the assessor wrote a description of the patient's changes and current situation.

While this interview took place the research assistant again talked with the informant, the patient's close friend or relative. She administered the SSIAM and they both rated the patient's work, social, sexual, and overall adjustment on thirteen-point comparative scales.

After these interviews, the research assistant gave both the patient and the informant packets of forms to be filled out at home and mailed back. The informant answered the "inquiry." The patient answered the "inquiry," the "checklist," and, if he had received treatment, the Truax Relationship Questionnaire and the Lorr Inventory. The latter two rating scales were used to measure the patient's attitude toward the therapist and the patient's perception of the therapist's behavior.

Therapists rated work, social, sexual, and overall change on a thirteen-point comparative scale, and also completed a scale designed to measure their attitude toward each patient.

# 4 Outcome of Treatment at Four Months

In this chapter group differences in outcome of treatment at four months are presented. We used as principal measures of outcome the changes in severity of the three target symptoms and changes in general adjustment level.

## TARGET SYMPTOMS

Ratings of the severity of the three target symptoms were made by assessors on a five-point scale at the initial, four-month, and one-year assessments. Mean assessor ratings of each of the three target symptoms at initial and four-month assessments are shown for each treatment group in Figure 1. These symptoms showed a similar pattern of change. All three groups began treatment with symptoms rated moderate in severity. Both actively treated groups decreased an average of one and one-half scale points, so that symptoms came between the "mild" and "trivial" points at four months. Wait list patients decreased only one-half scale point with symptoms rated between mild and moderate in severity. However, the improvement shown by all three groups for all three symptoms combined was statistically significant when tested by *t* tests.

Differences between treatment groups in degree of severity

Figure 1

Severity of Target Symptoms at Initial and Four-Month Assessment: Rated by Assessors

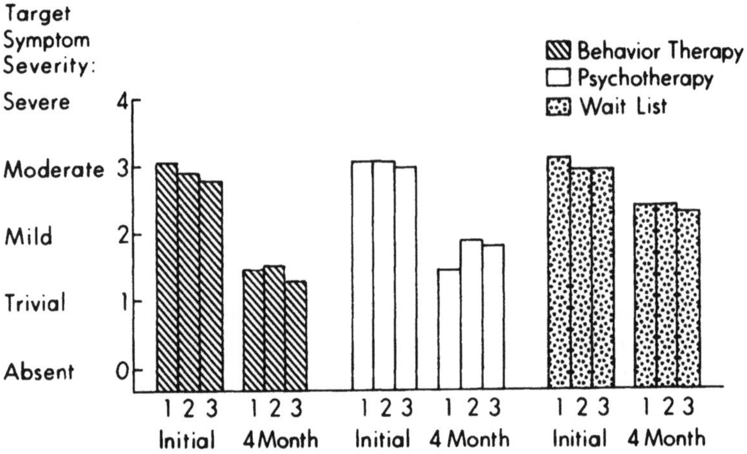


reduction, tested by means of multivariate analysis of variance, are shown in Table 8. Patients treated by behavior therapy clearly showed significantly greater improvement than wait list patients across all three target symptoms and in each of the three symptoms taken separately. Similarly, patients treated by psychotherapy showed greater improvement than wait list patients on the multivariate comparison and on each of the three individual symptoms. Differences between the two treated groups did not approach statistical significance for individual or multivariate comparisons. Thus, patients treated by behavior therapy and by psychotherapy improved equally in all three of their target symptoms after four months' treatment, and significantly more than the wait-list patients did.

In terms of symptomatic change, then, all three groups were

TABLE 8. Univariate and Multivariate F Values of Target Symptom Change

| Treatment Group | Symptom 1 | Symptom 2 | Symptom 3 | Multivariate |
|---|---|---|---|---|
| Behavior therapy vs. wait list | 9.0148[a] | 8.0513[a] | 9.5708[a] | 4.9292[a] |
| Psychotherapy vs. wait list | 12.1725[a] | 6.7628[b] | 4.6018[c] | 4.5742[b] |
| Behavior therapy vs. psychotherapy | .2374 | .0563 | .9027 | .5184 |

[a] $p < .005$
[b] $p < .01$
[c] $p < .05$

significantly improved, with both actively treated groups showing a similar pattern of improvement which was significantly greater than that of wait-list patients.

## GENERAL FUNCTIONING LEVEL

A second measure of response to therapy involved changes in general personality functioning in areas not necessarily connected with the three main target symptoms. The Structured and Scaled Interview to Assess Maladjustment (SSIAM) was used for this purpose. It will be recalled that the SSIAM consists of items grouped under five main areas including work, social and leisure life, sexual adjustment, family of origin, and marriage adjustment. The SSIAM has proved a reliable and useful instrument to measure degree of pathology. Gurland and his colleagues performed a varimax factor analysis of 33 of the 45 items (those which were completed for the majority of the patients) on ratings obtained from 164 adults accepted for outpatient psychotherapy.[1] This standardization sample consisted of patients from the present study and a second group of similar patients from the Johns Hopkins Outpatient Clinic. The analysis yielded six major factors labeled: social isolation, work inadequacy, friction with family, dependence on family, sexual dissatisfaction, and friction outside family. These factors are relatively independent and show a high degree of interrater agreement.[2]

However, several problems were encountered in using this instrument as a measure of change. First was the problem of missing data. This was most evident in the areas of sexual adjustment and also marriage. Obviously the whole section on marriage was not completed for those who were single. For those with little or no experience in sexual intercourse, the items in the sexual area were largely not applicable. A second problem involved the legitimacy of using certain items which could not reasonably be expected to show change after four months of treatment. Such items were often in the area of family of origin. Many patients, particularly students, were living away from home and had little or no contact with their family during the period of treatment. Therefore, it was not felt to be appropriate to use items such as, "Are there members of your family in whom you confide?" or "How do you get along with your family?" as indicators of change for patients who have little or no opportunity to modify these activities during the treatment period.

As a result it was decided to use the first two major factors from the analysis, "work inadequacy" and "social isolation," as measures of response to treatment. All items comprising the social factor and four of the five items comprising the work factor were completed by the majority of patients and considered valid indicators of change. The items with their factor loadings are:

| *Social Isolation* | | *Factor Loading* |
|---|---|---|
| S1 | Isolated. Are you keeping in touch with friends? | .61 |
| S7 | Distressed by company. Are you ill at ease, tense, shy or upset when with friends? | .48 |
| S9 | Bored by leisure. Do you often feel bored when not working? | .45 |
| S8 | Lonely. Do you feel the need for more companionship? | .43 |
| S2 | Constrained. Are you being open about your feelings in talking to friends? | .34 |
| *Work Inadequacy* | | |
| W2 | Inefficient. How well do you do your work? | .68 |
| W9 | Feeling inadequate. Do you feel inferior at work? Do you feel your work has proved worthwhile? | .57 |

| *Work Inadequacy* | | *Factor Loading* |
|---|---|---|
| W3 | Unsuccessful. Are you making progress in your work or career? | .48 |
| W7 | Disinterested. Do you find your work interesting? | .36 |

Mean scores were taken for each subject for each factor.

Mean factor scores for work inadequacy and social isolation at initial and four-month assessments are plotted graphically for each treatment group in Figure 2. For work inadequacy, the difference between initial and four-month assessments was highly significant in the case of the behavior therapy group ($p < .001$), suggesting that patients treated by behavior therapy showed a decrease in severity of work pathology with their course of treatment. Although both the psychotherapy and the wait list groups showed improvement, the improvement was only marginally significant. That is, it was significant when a one-tailed test was used but not when a two-tailed test was used. See Appendix 4 for a discussion of levels of significance and *t* tests. There is some controversy in the statistical literature concerning the appropriateness of two-tailed vs. one-tailed tests of significance.

Behavior therapy patients showed significant improvement in social adjustment ($p < .05$), as did patients who were on the wait list during this period ($P < .01$). Patients treated by pyschotherapy were not significantly different at the four-month assessment than at initial assessment. The largest change shown was one full scale point (from 4 to 3) by the behavior therapy group on work adjustment. While this indicated a consistent and significant improvement, it did not reflect the major shift which seemed clinically apparent. This was no doubt due at least in part to outpatients' tendency to cluster toward the lower (better adjusted) end of the scale, leaving relatively little room for measurable improvement.

Figure 2

SSIAM Work and Social Pathology at Initial and Four-Month Assessment: Rated by Assessors

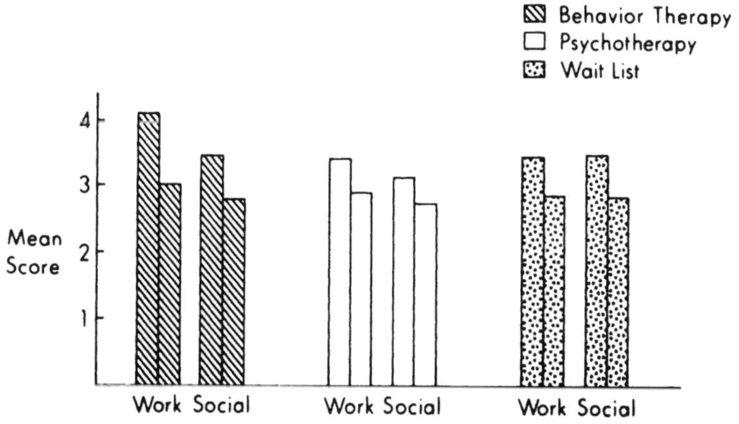


Comparisons of amount of improvement in work and social adjustment, and in symptomatic improvement, were tested in 3 x 2 x 2 analyses of variance with treatment as one factor, patient sex as the second, and severity of neuroticism as the third factor. As can be seen in Table 9, between-group differences in amount of improvement did not approach statistical significance for either work or social adjustment. Neither of the active treatment groups showed a significantly greater improvement than wait list patients on either measure when individual comparisons were made by $t$ tests. There were no significant differences in improvement between those who were severely and moderately neurotic, or between males and females. None of the interactions with type of treatment approached statistical significance for target symptoms, work, or social adjustment. The improvement shown at four months, then, appears to be independent of sex and degree of neuroticism as measured by the Eysenck Personality Inventory.

TABLE 9. Analyses of Variance of Four-Month Change Scores

| | | Work Inadequacy | | Social Isolation | | Target Symptoms | |
|---|---|---|---|---|---|---|---|
| Source | df | M.S. | F | M.S. | F | M.S. | F |
| Treatments | 2 | 3.44 | 1.46 | 1.16 | .55 | 60.03 | 9.95[a] |
| Neuroticism | 1 | 4.33 | 1.85 | .21 | .10 | 8.71 | 1.44 |
| Sex | 1 | .27 | .11 | 2.43 | 1.15 | .13 | .02 |
| Treatments X neuroticism | 2 | .71 | .30 | 3.79 | 1.80 | .88 | .13 |
| Treatments X sex | 2 | 2.32 | .99 | .36 | .17 | 4.47 | .74 |
| Neuroticism X sex | 1 | .31 | .13 | .49 | .23 | 1.03 | .17 |
| Treatments X sex X neuroticism | 2 | 1.72 | .73 | 4.45 | 2.11 | 6.38 | 1.06 |
| Error | 78 | 2.35 | | 2.11 | | 6.03 | |
| Total | 89 | | | | | | |

[a] $p < .001$

In summary, patients treated by behavior therapy and psychotherapy showed significantly greater reduction in the severity of their target symptoms than did patients on the wait list control. All groups showed significant improvement over their pre-treatment condition. However, the greater symptomatic relief of patients receiving active treatment was not associated with greater improvement in their work and social life. Wait-list patients showed improvement equal to that of the behavior therapy and psychotherapy patients on these measures. Patients' sex and initial neuroticism level also had no significant direct effect on amount of improvement; nor did these factors influence the effectiveness of the different treatments.

## THERAPIST EXPERIENCE AND OUTCOME

Therapists in both active treatment groups can conveniently be grouped in three levels of experience in dealing with neurotic patients. Did amount of previous experience have an effect on treatment outcome, particularly for those patients who are severely neurotic? It might be expected that therapists with greater experience would be more effective in the management of severely ill patients than would their less experienced colleagues.

A 2 x 3 x 2 analysis of variance with treatments (behavior therapy versus psychotherapy), therapist experience (high, medium, and low), and degree of neuroticism (moderate versus severe) was performed on each improvement measure for those patients in the two active treatment groups (Table 10). Patients treated by less experienced therapists showed improvement on all measures equal to those treated by more experienced therapists. Therapists in both active treatment groups appeared to do equally well with severely and moderately neurotic patients.

It should be recalled, however, that the level of experience in the present study is considerably higher than in most investigations. All therapists had treated neurotic patients for some time. The two least experienced had seen approximately three hundred patients during the past six years. The comparison here might more properly be regarded as between qualified therapists of varying experience, rather than between expert and inexperienced or beginning therapists.

The nonsignificant interaction terms for treatments x experience also indicate that all six therapists were equally effective in treating patients. The observed treatment effects are not solely due to the efforts of one or two therapists in each group.

TABLE 10. Analyses of Variance of Four-Month Change Scores: Patients in Active Treatment Groups

| | | Target Symptoms | | Work Inadequacy | | Social Isolation | |
|---|---|---|---|---|---|---|---|
| Source | df | M.S. | F | M.S. | F | M.S. | F |
| Treatments | 1 | .02 | .00 | 6.50 | 3.44 | .86 | .37 |
| Therapist experience | 2 | 1.95 | .26 | 2.28 | 1.21 | 2.67 | 1.16 |
| Neuroticism | 1 | 2.82 | .38 | 5.55 | 2.94 | 1.06 | .46 |
| Treatments × experience | 2 | 2.12 | .29 | 4.54 | 2.40 | .21 | .09 |
| Treatments × neuroticism | 1 | .15 | .02 | .13 | .07 | 8.97 | 3.88 |
| Experience × neuroticism | 2 | 1.02 | .14 | .01 | .01 | 1.24 | .54 |
| Treatments × neuroticism × experience | 2 | .05 | .01 | 4.48 | 2.37 | .49 | .21 |
| Error | 48 | 7.38 | | 1.89 | | 2.31 | |
| Total | 59 | | | | | | |

## ANXIETY AS A SYMPTOM

Many writers consider anxiety the essential characteristic of neurosis. Because of this, we separately compared the three treatments for their success in reducing anxiety. The assessor rated severity of anxiety at the initial assessment and at the four-month interview on the same five-point scale used for target symptoms. If some form of anxiety was not listed as one of the three target symptoms, a separate rating was taken. A change or improvement score was taken for each patient by subtracting the post-treatment rating from the pre-treatment rating.

Overall, 61% of the patients showed a trend toward improvement in anxiety during the treatment period (Figure 3). Fewer of the patients on the wait list showed an improvement (53%) than either the behavior therapy (66%) or psychotherapy (63%) groups, although these differences did not reach statistical significance ( $\chi^2 = 1.2152$). To test for differences in the amount of improvement between different groups, a 2 x 2 x 3 analysis of variance was used with degree of neuroticism, sex of patient, and method of treatment as factors (Table 11). The main effects for treatment did not reach statistical significance, suggesting no overall difference among behavior therapy, psychotherapy, or wait list patients in reduction of anxiety. There was a significant main effect for sex, with female patients showing more improvement than males. However, the treatments x severity x sex interaction term also reached statistical significance, suggesting that the greater improvement shown by females was not consistent for different neuroticism levels and treatment conditions.

We separately examined change scores for the patients in the two treated groups in order to test for differences related to therapist experience level and possible interactions between the individual therapist and patient personality characteristics

Figure 3

Change in Anxiety at Four Months: Rated by Assessors

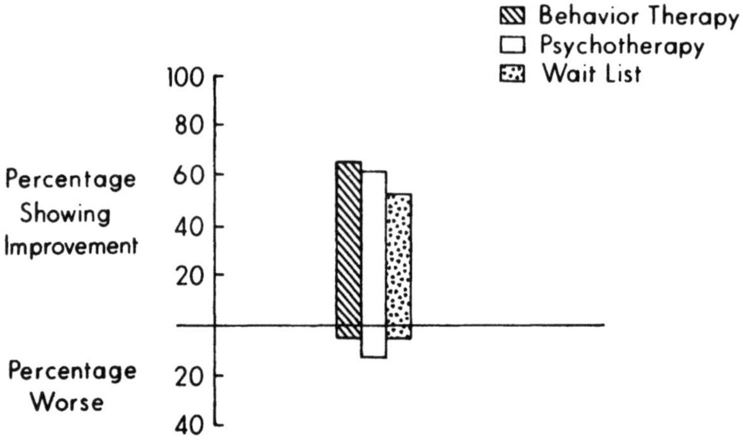


(Table 11). Analysis of variance indicated no difference between treatments. Level of therapist experience appeared to have no effect on amount of anxiety reduction. While there was a tendency for highly neurotic patients to show more improvement, this trend did not reach statistical significance, nor were any of the interaction terms significant.

The effect of treatment on anxiety was tested regardless of whether or not anxiety caused the patient much distress. For some patients, a reduction of severity of anxiety might not be particularly therapeutic or a valid test of the treatment. Consequently, we separately examined those patients who reported some form of anxiety as one of their three target symptoms.

There was some tendency for patients treated by psychotherapy to show greater improvement, although this trend did not reach statistical significance ($F = 3.2524$; $p < .10$).

TABLE 11. Changes in Anxiety at Four Months: Analyses of Variance

| All Patients | | | |
|---|---|---|---|
| Source | df | M.S. | F |
| Treatments | 2 | .88 | .97 |
| Neuroticism | 1 | 1.11 | 1.23 |
| Sex | 1 | 11.27 | 12.44[a] |
| Treatments X neuroticism | 2 | .68 | .75 |
| Treatments X sex | 2 | .62 | .69 |
| Neuroticism X sex | 1 | .19 | .20 |
| Treatmentx X sex X neuroticism | 2 | 3.79 | 4.18[b] |
| Error | 78 | .91 | |
| Total | 89 | | |

| Treated Patients Only | | | |
|---|---|---|---|
| Source | df | M.S. | F |
| Treatments | 1 | .07 | .05 |
| Therapist experience | 2 | .07 | .05 |
| Neuroticism | 1 | 2.40 | 1.89 |
| Treatments X experience | 2 | .47 | .37 |
| Treatments X neuroticism | 1 | .60 | .47 |
| Experience X neuroticism | 2 | .20 | .16 |
| Treatments X experience X neuroticism | 2 | .20 | .16 |
| Error | 48 | 1.27 | |
| Total | 59 | | |

[a]$p < .001$
[b]$p < .05$

## SYMPTOM SUBSTITUTION

During the four-month reassessment interview, any new symptoms were noted and rated in the usual way by the assessor. These were not subjected to any formal analysis but were useful evidence of the symptom substitution expected by some authorities to occur when a symptom is quickly and superficially removed without longer treatment to remove its underlying causes.

A few patients who had not improved in four months reported additional symptoms which either were new or had been too trivial to report at initial assessment. However, there was not a single patient in any group whose original problems had substantially improved but who reported new symptoms cropping up. On the contrary, assessors had the informal impression that when a patient's primary symptoms improved, he often spontaneously reported improvement of other minor difficulties.

In short, in this sample we had no evidence whatsoever of symptom substitution.

## PERCENTAGE OF PATIENTS IMPROVED

Psychotherapy studies have typically included a report of the percentage of patients who improve and those who do not, including the percentage of those considered cured. Such ratings are presented below, to aid in cross comparison among studies by providing a more traditional representation of therapeutic outcome. At four months assessors rated improvement in overall adjustment and target symptoms on similar thirteen-point scales. In order to report the percentages in more convenient categories consistent with other reports, the thirteen-point scale was collapsed to five points as shown.

Thirteen-point scale

| | | | | |
|---|---|---|---|---|
| 0 1 | 2 3 4 | 5 6 7 | 8 9 10 | 11 12 |
| very much worse | much worse / a little worse | no change | a little better / much better | completely recovered |

| | | | | |
|---|---|---|---|---|
| very much worse | worse | no change | improved | completely recovered |
| 0 | 1 | 2 | 3 | 4 |

Five-point scale

The anchoring-point definitions of the overall adjustment and target symptom severity scales were identical.

Figure 4 shows the percentage of patients in each group who were rated by the assessor as very much worse, worse, showing no change, improved, or completely recovered in terms of their target symptoms. Only one patient was considered worse symptomatically. This person was in the wait-list group. Eighty percent of the patients in each of the active treatment groups were considered either improved or recovered, significantly higher than the 48 percent improved or recovered in the wait-list group ($\chi^2 = 9.31$; $p < .01$). Improvement rates for overall adjustment tended to be higher than for symptomatic change (Figure 5). Ninety-three percent of the patients treated by behavior therapy were considered improved while 77 percent of both psychotherapy and wait-list patients were either improved or recovered ($\chi^2 = 3.93$; $p < .05$). Two patients were felt to have deteriorated overall during the four-month period, one in psychotherapy and one in the wait-list group. Curiously, two wait-list patients but no

Figure 4

Target Symptom Severity at Four Months: Rated by Assessors

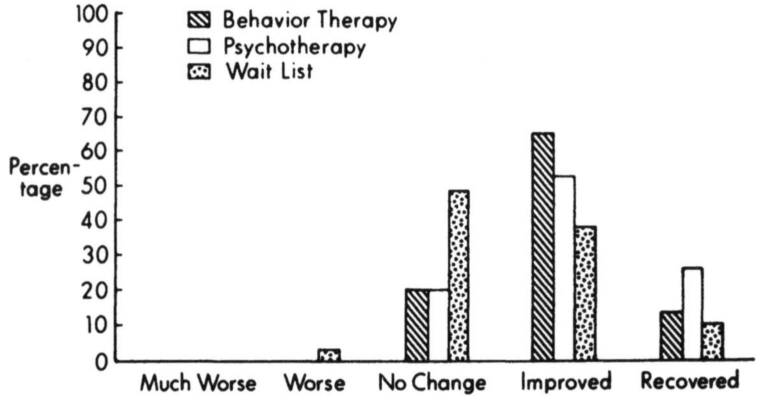


Figure 5

Overall Adjustment at Four Months: Rated by Assessors

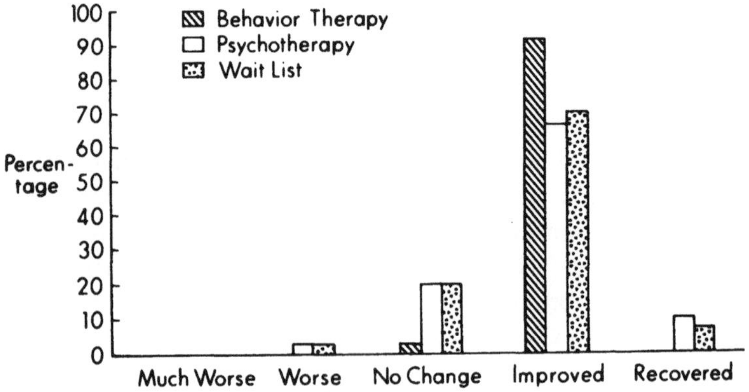

behavior therapy patients were considered completely recovered.

Therapeutic gains seen by the assessors in the present study were equal to if not greater than the improvement rates claimed by proponents of the two active treatments. Results also compared favorably with the improvement rates of previous outcome studies summarized by Bergin.[3] Thus the treatment was successful. The lack of greater overall differences between the treated and untreated patients appeared due to the impressive 77% improvement of the untreated, in contrast to Bergin's reported median of 30% improvement in untreated control groups.

This highlights the necessity of matching treated and untreated patients in any study of psychotherapy. Uncontrolled factors vary so much from one study to another that it is difficult to compare a treated group's improvement with some abstract summary of the "improvement of untreated patients." Ninety-three percent of behavior therapy patients improved overall. This figure would have seemed not merely significant, but downright miraculous, if it were compared to Bergin's 30% figure, rather than to the 77% improvement this sample actually showed without formal treatment.

## PATIENT PERCEPTIONS OF TREATMENT

Thus far we have focused on the asssessors' independent ratings of improvement. The opinions of the patients themselves have not been heard. At the four-month and one-year assessments, patients rated their improvement on thirteen-point scales similar to the assessor ratings described earlier. For purposes of illustrating the effect of therapy in terms of percentage of patients showing change, the scale was again collapsed to five points.

Figure 6 shows the percentage of patients who considered

Figure 6

Change in Target Symptoms at Four Months: Rated by Patient

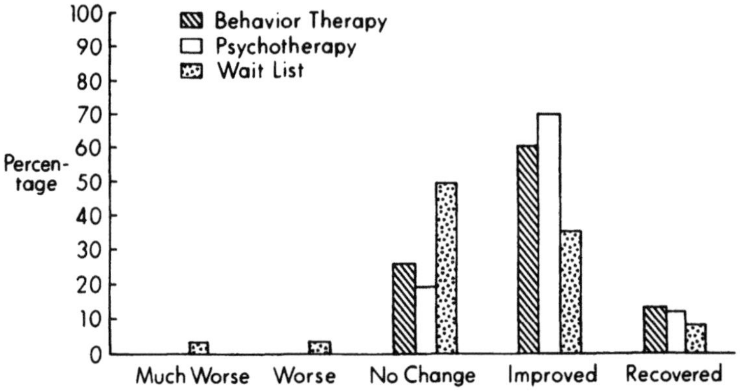


their target symptoms to be much worse, worse, the same, improved, or completely recovered at four months. Only two patients, both in the wait-list group, felt their symptoms were either worse or much worse. Few (less than 15% in any group) felt their original problems were now recovered. More patients in both active treatment groups than on the wait list felt they had improved or recovered ($\chi^2 = 8.59$; $p < .05$). Seventy-four percent of behavior therapy and 81% of psychotherapy patients rated themselves as improved or recovered, in contrast to less than half (44%) of wait-list patients. These figures are remarkably similar to the 80%, 80%, and 48% symptomatic improvement rates judged by the assessors, and indicate considerable agreement between patient and assessor points of view.

We can also compare patient and assessor ratings of overall adjustment at four months. Significantly more patients in the active treatment groups than on the wait list considered themselves either improved or recovered ($\chi^2 = 10.50$; $p < .05$).

Ninety-three percent of behavior therapy and 80% of psychotherapy patients felt they had benefited from their treatment. The only marked difference between patient and assessor ratings appeared to be for those on the wait list; the 55% "improved" self-rating by patients (Figure 7) contrasts with the assessor rating of 77% (Figure 5). It seems understandable that patients who were still waiting for a promised treatment might consider themselves worse than an observer would.

We also compared group ratings of improvement in work, social, and sexual adjustment. Figure 8 shows the mean patient ratings at four months for each of these measures, as well as target symptom severity and overall adjustment. These data are derived from the original thirteen-point rating scale. Point six represents "no change", eight represents "a little better" and ten represents "much better". Both treated groups tended to show similar average improvement which is consistently greater than that of wait-list patients. However, analyses of variance (Tables 12 and 13) indicate that only on tar-

Figure 7

Overall Improvement at Four Months: Rated by Patient

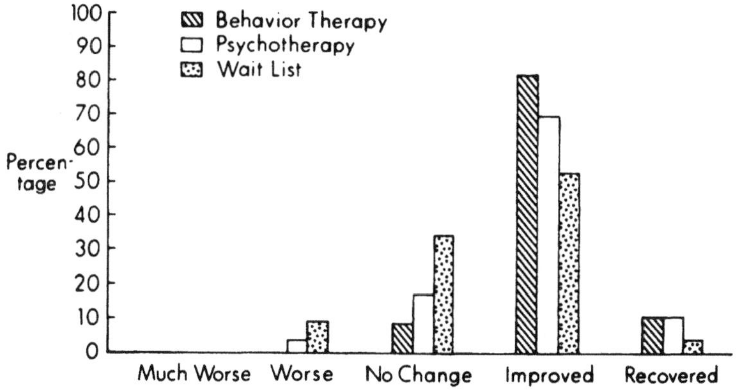

TABLE 12. Target Symptom Severity and Overall Adjustment at Four Months: Analyses of Variance of Patient Comparative Ratings

| | Target Symptoms | | | Overall Adjustment | | |
|---|---|---|---|---|---|---|
| Source | df | M.S. | F | df | M.S. | F |
| Treatments | 2 | 121.92 | 4.05[a] | 2 | 9.71 | 2.98 |
| Within groups | 72 | 30.09 | | 84 | 3.26 | |
| Total | 74 | | | 86 | | |

[a] $p < .05$

TABLE 13. Work, Social, and Sexual Adjustment at Four Months: Analyses of Variance of Patient Comparative Ratings

| | Work Adjustment | | | Social Adjustment | | | Sexual Adjustment | | |
|---|---|---|---|---|---|---|---|---|---|
| Source | df | M.S. | F | df | M.S. | F | df | M.S. | F |
| Treatments | 2 | 12.15 | 2.79 | 2 | 1.85 | .38 | 2 | 20.30 | 3.56[a] |
| Within groups | 66 | 4.36 | | 67 | 4.89 | | 70 | 5.70 | |
| Total | 68 | | | 69 | | | 72 | | |

[a] $p < .05$

get symptoms did both treated groups rate themselves as significantly more improved than wait-list patients. Furthermore, psychotherapy patients rated themselves as significantly more improved on sexual adjustment than either of the other two groups (See Figure 8 and Table 13).

Conclusions drawn from this analysis of group patient ratings are similar to the principal outcome ratings by assessors. Both treated groups showed greater symptomatic improvement, but there were no differences among the three groups in work, social, or overall adjustment. Sexual adjustment, in the patients' opinion, was helped more by psychotherapy than by behavior therapy or the wait-list regimen.

Figure 8

Improvement at Four Months, by area: Rated by Patient

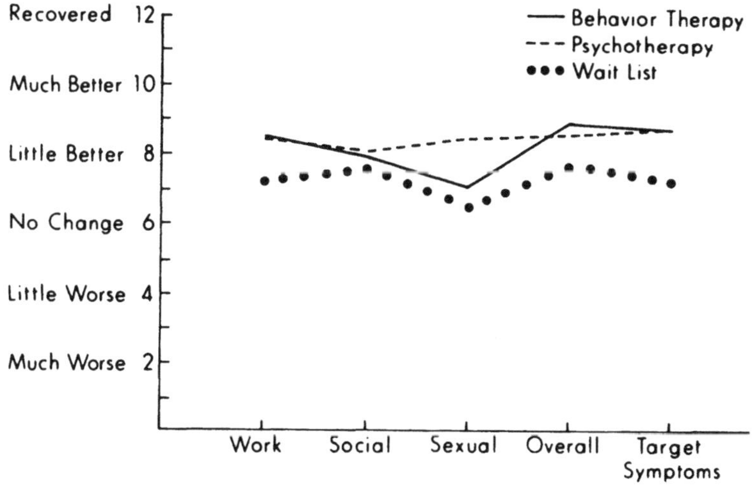


## COMPARISON OF DIFFERENT RATERS

Psychotherapy studies have sometimes used more than one source of information about the outcome of treatment. Outcome may be assessed by an independent professional evaluator, by the therapist, the patient, or some outside source, such as a friend or relative of the patient. In the present study we wished to compare the estimates obtained from each of these sources, in order to provide a more valid basis of comparison among studies which have used some of these outcome criteria. A second aim was to see how different people perceive changes in the patient. The therapist, the independent assessor, the patient, and the friend or relative (informant), each has a unique vantage point from which to view the effects of treatment. Each may have distinctive, private goals for treatment which differ from others' goals. A therapist may see vast improvement where the patient's wife sees dismal failure.

Both the patient and the therapist have invested considerable time, effort, and energy in the treatment process. The patient has come for evaluation, has gone through a battery of tests, and has appeared for treatment weekly for a period of four months. The therapist has invested years of training, as well as time spent with the individual patient. Consequently, both have committed themselves emotionally and intellectually to the treatment process and they may strongly resist admitting failure. Patients also differ in their attitude toward treatment, expectations of what might be accomplished, feelings of attraction or dislike toward the therapist. Such factors may influence judgment of the effects of treatment.

The assessments of an independent psychiatrist and an informant would seem to be more objective sources of information. The assessor might be biased toward one or another treatment and expect more improvement from treated than from nontreated patients. However, our assessors were surprisingly successful in remaining blind to the type of treatment a patient received. In addition, since he is not intimately involved in the therapeutic process, the assessor can still retain considerable objectivity as an independent observer. The informant stands somewhere between the assessor and the patient in degree of independence of the treatment. While by definition there is a positive relationship with the patient and a desire to see improvement, relatives are at the same time notorious for resisting change in patients. Still, informants are not as emotionally committed to treatment as are patients and therefore are not open to the same source of bias.

At the time of the four-month assessment, patients were rated by the assessor, informant, therapist, and themselves on work, social, sexual, and overall adjustment relative to their status at initial assessment on the same thirteen-point scale. Raters were instructed not to guess at changes unless they had sufficient information to make a valid judgment. Thus, the mother of a male patient might not have adequate information on changes in the patient's sexual life, and consequently she was asked to complete only the ratings for work, social, and overall adjustment. This restriction, combined with the failure of several informants to return for the four-month interview, severely limited the number of patients for whom complete ratings were available. However, we felt the procedure to be justified since we wanted to compare different raters' clear, definite perceptions.

Mean values of comparative ratings of change by the assessor, patient, informant, and therapist for work, social, and sexual adjustment are shown in Figures 9, 10, and 11. These figures are based on data from those patients who had complete ratings in a given area of adjustment from all possible raters.

Figure 9

Different Raters' Estimates of Improvement for Behavior Therapy Patients

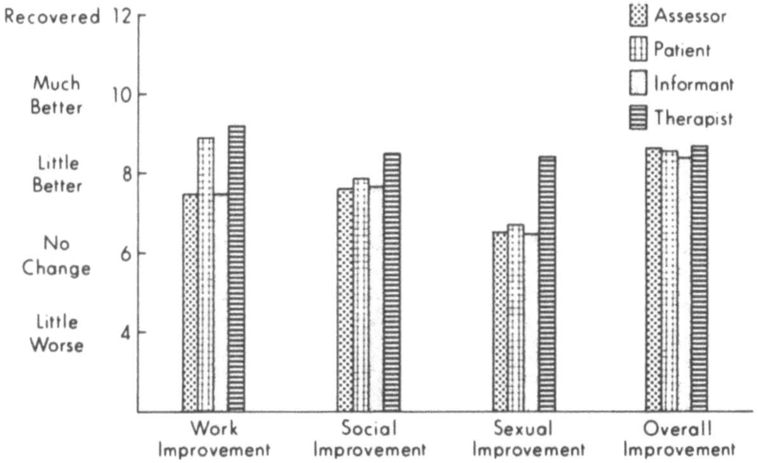

**Figure 10**

**Different Raters' Estimates of Improvement for Psychotherapy Patients**

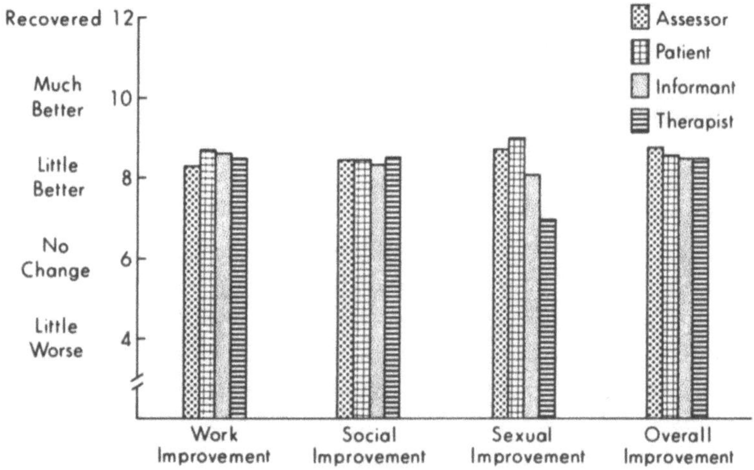


Figure 11

Different Raters' Estimates of Improvement for Wait List Patients

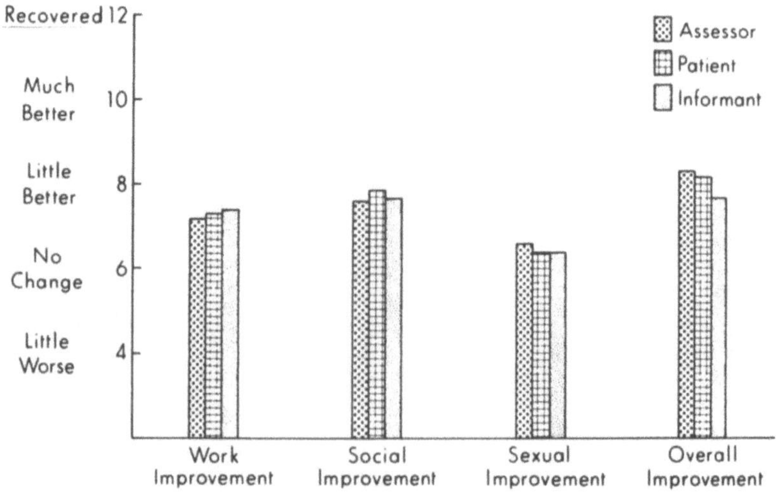

Differences among raters in each area were tested for statistical significance by analysis of variance (repeated-measures-on-the-same-subject design). Individual comparisons following significant analyses of variance were tested by means of Duncan's Multiple Range Test.

There were no significant differences among raters in work adjustment for patients treated by psychotherapy or for wait-list patients. There was, in fact, considerable agreement among raters with psychotherapy patients consistently considered somewhat more than a little better (8), and wait-list patients showing slight improvement (7). However, there was considerable variability among raters in assessing patients treated by behavior therapy ($F = 3.68$; $p < .05$). Behavior therapists rated their patients as showing significantly greater improvement than did assessors or informants ($p < .05$). This represents a difference of nearly two scale points. Patient ratings were most similar to those of the therapists, although not significantly different from assessors or informants.

Ratings of improvement in social adjustment were more consistent than in work adjustment. There were no significant differences among raters for any group except that behavior therapists tended to rate their patients as showing greater improvement than other raters.

Both groups of therapists tended to give idiosyncratic ratings of sexual adjustment. Behavior therapists once again rated their patients as showing greater improvement than did assessors, patients, or informants ($F = 3.50$; $p < .05$). Psychotherapists tended to perceive less improvement in their patients than did other observers, although this trend did not reach statistical significance ($F = 2.43$; $p < .10$). Even so, the mean difference between psychotherapist and patient ratings were nearly two full scale points, similar to the discrepancy in behavior therapy. Wait-list patients were considered to show a similar degree of improvement by all raters.

While there was considerable agreement among raters, therapist ratings tended to be somewhat deviant. To further explore these relationships, single improvement scores were taken for each rater by summing the ratings for work, social, and sexual improvement for each patient. Scores were then intercorrelated. As might be expected from the comparison of the group means, ratings made by therapists did not correlate highly with those of the other evaluators.

Correlations of therapist scores were .13, .21, and −.04 with ratings made by assessors, patients, and informants respectively. These correlations indicate little relationship and suggest that outcome ratings made by the therapist cannot be substituted for ratings made by the assessor, patient, or informant with any assurance that similar results will emerge.

Ratings made by the assessor show considerable concordance with those of the patient ($r = .65$; $p < .001$), and to a lesser extent with those of the informant ($r = .40$; $p < .01$). There is much less agreement between patient and informant ($r = .25$). These relatively low correlations support the hypothesis that different raters may have different goals for treatment or use different criteria for improvement. Even though the average degree of improvement for a group may be similar for two raters, the low intercorrelations indicate that a patient considered improved by one rater may not be the same patient considered improved by the second rater. This further underscores the hazard of interpreting similar group means as reflecting similar perception of individuals.

## CASE HISTORIES

The following summaries are illustrative of changes which took place in patients during treatment. All these patients were described in Chapter Three as they appeared on admission.

Evelyn Ashley, the tense college senior who had used fantasy to withdraw from reality, improved remarkably after four months of psychotherapy. She said her psychotherapist had helped her to feel she was a decent person. She came to insist that her boyfriend respect her or else she would leave him; his attitude changed and their relationship improved tremendously. Her tension was much improved, and her feelings of inadequacy and retreating into fantasy were completely recovered. All these problems had been of very long standing. Her friendships had improved, and her sexual life was much more pleasurable. Evelyn's fiancé told the research assistant that she was much better, daydreamed much less, and was much less "lazy". Overall, she was very much improved.

"Things are an awful lot better. I feel very fortunate in having my doctor. My voice lessons have been going fantastically well." This represented the change in Marie Sutton after four months' psychotherapy. She had never expected to improve and was astonished at her own progress. Her feeling that she was about to pass out, which had persisted for several years prior to therapy, had been completely gone for three months, her extreme tension was almost gone, and she could concentrate very much better. The only residual problem was her boyfriend, whom she had not discussed with her therapist. She could see no future with him. After fifteen sessions of therapy she was rated much better overall.

After four months on the waiting list, Emma Hubbard was virtually unchanged. She still weighed 225 pounds. She had left home for the summer to work at the shore, and her social life and self-consciousness very slightly improved when she escaped from her domineering mother. She was now socializing with boys in a large group but still did not date. She was assigned to a senior resident for psychotherapy.

Tom Morton, the bearded premed student, was "ecstatic" at his four-month interview about his behavior therapy. He liked his therapist's philosophy of life and this helped to crystallize his own. His loneliness, lack of values, and need to impress people as tops had all just about disappeared. He had moved away from home. There remained some imperfections in his sexual life, but these struck the assessor as being less Tom's problem than his girlfriend's. He was much improved overall, but his mother told the research assistant that he had not changed and was very hyperactive.

After four months of psychotherapy, Raymond Simpson's tension, facial twitching, and feelings of inferiority remained. His depression had grown slightly worse, he was working less than before, and he had begun to eat "compulsively", whenever he was nervous. He was gaining weight and developing a flabby stomach. His relationship with his girlfriend was still satisfying to him, and his relationship with his father had improved considerably, but he felt this was coincidental to therapy.

After four months of psychotherapy, the black social worker, Veneta Williams was "immensely improved", according to her assessor, especially in terms of work. She had lost her depression, jitteriness, and feelings of suspicion and inadequacy at work. Her deeper character problems remained, with distant relationships to family and friends, but her immediate problems were much improved. Her brother told the research assistant that he had noticed no change in the patient since therapy began.

Norman Rollins had lost his pinched look at reassessment; he was visibly more relaxed and seemed actually to have gained weight. He admired his psychotherapist tremendously. He still had intermittent tension but had lost his constant anxiety in social situations, and all his target symptoms were much better. He asserted himself more, felt less guilt, and was sexually more comfortable and desirous. He had made definite plans for improving his career by attending a school of social work, with alternative plans if this should fall through. All in all, he described enormous improvement in every area of his life. His wife, on the other hand, told the research assistant that there had been no change whatever in Norman.

Louise Shaw's fear of incontinence had considerably improved after four months of behavior therapy, as had her other fears and anxieties. She still had difficulty in going out shopping, with occasional bad days when her fear returned, but her good days were now much more frequent. Her target symptoms were all rated between a little better and much better, and her husband thought she was a little better overall.

After four months' psychotherapy, Mary Teresa Moore had completely lost her obsessive thoughts about harming her children or herself. Her depression and anxiety were nearly gone, and in general she was almost completely recovered. She still felt a little guilt about sex but expected this to stop when she got married in three months, and she had a fine relationship with her fiancé. In summary, her rather severe symptoms had dramatically improved.

## CONCLUSIONS

At the end of the four-month treatment period, patients in all three groups showed considerable symptomatic improvement. Approximately fifty percent of the wait-list patients and eighty percent of the behavior therapy and psychotherapy patients were considered improved or recovered symptomatically. Patients treated by behavior therapy and psychotherapy did show more average symptomatic improvement than patients in the minimal treatment group. There were no differences between the two active treatment groups.

Improvement in work adjustment and social isolation was less consistent. Patients treated by behavior therapy showed significant improvement in both work and social adjustment, while psychotherapy patients showed only marginal improvement in work and no change in social adjustment. Wait-list patients showed significant improvement in social and marginal improvement in work adjustment. However, none of the between-group comparisons were statistically significant.

The amount of improvement shown appeared to be independent of the sex of the patient, severity of neurosis, and degree of therapist experience. The exception was that the anxiety of females (and especially high-neurotic females) improved more than males.

The majority of all three groups, but significantly more of the behavior therapy group, were judged "improved" or "recovered" on a global rating of improvement.

Improvement of wait-list patients was quite consistent, not only in symptomatic change but in work and social adjustment as well.

Patients' ratings of improvement accorded well with those of the assessors, both in improvement rates and in differences between groups. Ratings made by therapists appeared to deviate most from those of other observers. The highest correlations were shown by patient-assessor pairs, followed in decreasing order by assessor-informant, informant-patient, patient-therapist, therapist-assessor, and therapist-informant pairs.

# 5 Follow-Up Evaluations

Ideally, for research purposes, none of the patients would have received therapy between the four-month assessment and the one-year interview, but ethically we could not completely control treatment after the initial four-month period. In terms of our implicit contract with the patients, the decision to continue or terminate treatment was theirs alone. It had been suggested at the initial assessment that they should receive considerable benefit from four months' treatment. However, at the four month assessment treated patients had the option of continuing treatment with their current therapist (if he was willing), continuing with another therapist provided by the assessor, seeking a new therapist on their own, or terminating treatment altogether. Similarly, patients on the wait list were free to forgo formal therapy altogether or to be assigned a therapist provided by the assessor. All patients were assured that further treatment, if desired, was readily available. Thus, the comparison of the three forms of management becomes clouded after the initial four-month period. Nevertheless, there are obvious advantages to conducting follow-up investigations of these patients to trace their subsequent psychiatric history as closely as possible. Such investigations were made at one- and two-year intervals following initial assessment.

## ONE-YEAR REASSESSMENT

As close as possible to one year after the initial assessment, all but two of the original patients saw their original assessors once more, for an interview similar to the four-month reassessment. The actual time elapsed was somewhat greater than one year. Mean number of days between initial and one-year interviews was 392, 388, and 397 for the behavior therapy, psychotherapy, and wait list groups respectively. The two patients who were lost had both been rather early dropouts from behavior therapy. One felt he no longer wished to be in a research study; the other remained friendly and otherwise cooperative but was elusive and broke innumerable appointments without notice. Informal inquiry revealed that both had improved considerably by the one-year reassessment. Most patients were remarkably cooperative in coming for assessment interviews, and a great many expressed appreciation, not only for their therapy but also for the assessments themselves, which they had found rewarding and helpful.

The following measures were used at this reassessment:

1. Severity of target symptoms; absolute and comparative severity rated by assessor and patient.
2. SSIAM.
3. Comparative work, social, sexual, and overall adjustment rated by assessor and patient.
4. Anxiety, feeling at ease, disturbing events—the checklist of emotional symptoms.
5. A description of the kind and amount of therapy received since the four-month assessment.

Once again the research assistant interviewed the patient's close friend or relative. In several cases the informant had grown away from the patient or for other reasons could not be interviewed. Sometimes roommates had moved out of town, spouses had separated, children had moved away from home and lost touch with parents. Only thirty-one informant interviews could be completed at one year. The informant rated the patient's comparative work, social, sexual, and overall adjustment, and the SSIAM was conducted. Informants and patients were given forms to mail back: the "inquiry" for the informant and both the inquiry and the "checklist" for the patient.

## TREATMENT BETWEEN FOUR-MONTH AND ONE-YEAR ASSESSMENTS

The number of contacts with therapists during the ensuing eight-month period was determined by checking therapists' records and from patients' reports at the one-year interview. Both groups of therapists had some brief contact with patients during this period. Five behavior therapy and four psychotherapy patients were seen on one or two occasions. Such contacts were either highly informal—telephone calls or a visit to a patient while in a hospital for a medical problem—or else routine follow-up interviews occasioned by a period of stress in the patient's life. We did not consider them to represent further formal treatment.

However, a total of fifteen behavior therapy, nine psychotherapy, and twenty-two wait list patients had at least three therapy sessions during this period. Table 14 shows the number of visits to the same therapist for previously treated patients, and the type of new treatment received for those who saw new therapists. The three behavior therapy and four psychotherapy patients who saw new therapists were all treated by insight therapy, as were the majority of wait-list patients. Most of the new therapists provided by the assessors were senior psychiatric residents who were predominantly analytical in orientation.

## OUTCOME AT ONE YEAR

The pattern of change between four months and one year appeared to be a consolidation of improvement shown during the

TABLE 14. Patients Receiving Treatment Between Four-Month and One-Year Assessments

| Original Group | Type of Subsequent Treatment | Number of Visits 3-5 | 6-10 | 11-25 | 26+ | Total Number of Patients |
|---|---|---|---|---|---|---|
| Behavior therapy | Same therapist | 4 | 3 | 4 | 1 | 15 |
| | Psychotherapy | 1 | 2 | 0 | 0 | |
| Psycho-therapy | Same therapist | 0 | 1 | 1 | 3 | 9 |
| | Other Psycho-therapy | 0 | 0 | 4 | 0 | |
| Wait list | Behavior therapy | 0 | 1 | 1 | 1 | 22 |
| | Psychotherapy | 0 | 4 | 9 | 6 | |

first four months. Patients who were improved at four months tended to show continued improvement during the succeeding eight months. Only two patients who were improved symptomatically at four months were worse at one year, and these patients had shown only slight original improvement. Conversely, if improvement was not shown in the first four months, it was less likely to be shown at the one-year assessment, regardless of whether the patient had further treatment in the intervening period. Of the patients who did not show improvement at four months, 64% were still not improved on target symptoms, 70% on work adjustment, and 53% in their social adjustment, at one year. The initial four-month period would appear to be the critical time for change to occur.

Mean ratings of target symptom severity and work and social pathology at initial, four-month, and one-year assessments are shown for each of the three treatment groups in Figures 12, 13, and 14. Behavior therapy patients remained significantly improved over their initial status on all three measures. Psychotherapy patients continued improvement in social adjustment but were no longer significantly different from initial assessment in work adjustment. The 3 x 2 x 2 analyses of variance of these change scores with treatment groups, severity of neurosis, and sex of patient as factors are shown in Table 15. There were no overall differences among the three groups in amount of improvement on any of the three measures. None of the interaction terms involving treatment groups approached statistical significance. The only term which reached significance (sex x severity of neurosis on the SSIAM social factor) suggests that females of moderate pathology show less improvement in social functioning than do other patient subgroups. However, when differences between treatments were tested by individual *t* tests, patients in the behavior therapy group showed greater improvement on target symptoms than wait-list patients ($t = 2.1753$; $p < .05$). No other comparisons approached statistical significance.

Because of the complexity introduced by varying degrees of treatment between four months and one year, it is difficult to draw firm conclusions on the relative efficacy of the three forms of management at this time. Whatever improvement was evident one year after the original assessment might in part result from treatment received during this interval.

## TERMINATORS VERSUS CONTINUERS

A clearer comparison would involve only those patients who received no treatment following the four-month assessment. However, there are two problems in making a simple comparison of those patients. First, since these patients were "self-selected" rather than randomly assigned, it must be shown that patients in these three subgroups are similar to one another in the factors which may be related to amount of change shown. For example, patients in the wait-list group who showed con-

Figure 12

Target Symptom Severity: Assessor Ratings of All Patients

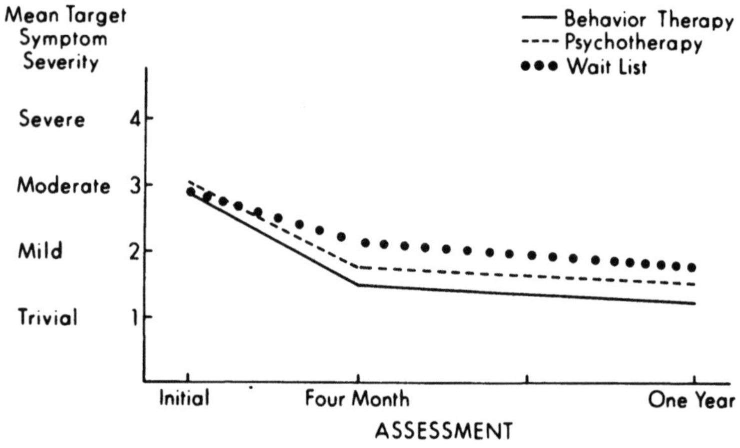


Figure 13

Work Inadequacy: Assessor SSIAM Ratings of All Patients

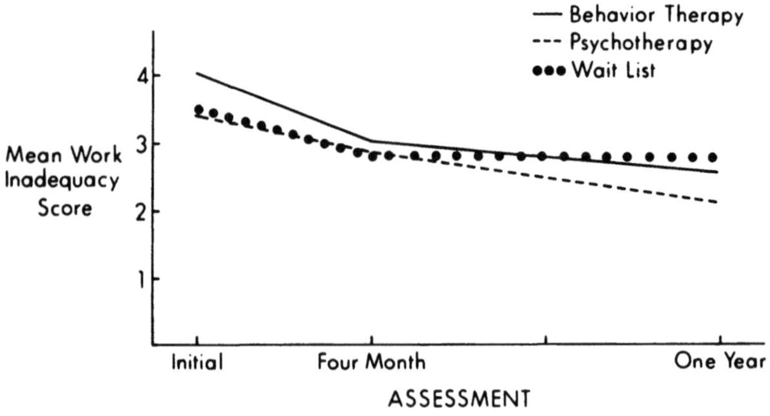

Figure 14

Social Isolation: Assessor SSIAM Ratings of All Patients

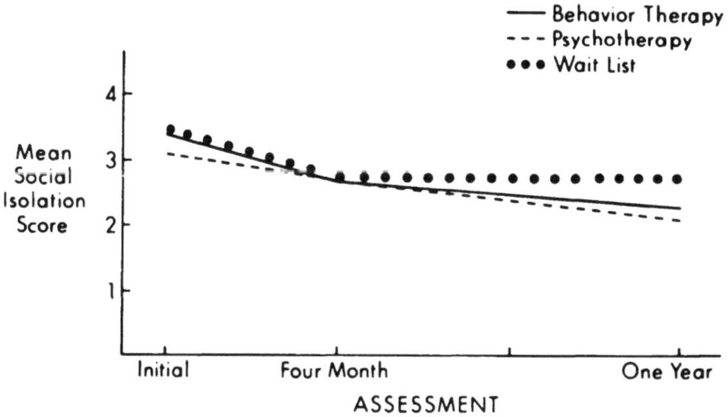


siderable improvement on their own by the time of the four-month assessment might decide not to accept treatment. Patients in one of the active treatment groups who received little benefit from therapy might also decide not to accept further treatment.

A comparison of subsequent improvement shown by two such groups of patients would not be a valid one. Secondly, if the results of the comparisons of patients who received no further treatment are to be generalized to the groups as a whole, it must be shown that the patients comprising these subgroups are representative of the patients in the full treatment groups. Consequently, the characteristics of those patients who did not seek further treatment were investigated in some detail.

The reasons for continuing or discontinuing therapy are complex and there did not appear to be a simple explanation for the choice. Several possibilities were examined:

1. One possibility was that patients who showed most im-

TABLE 15. Analyses of Variance of One-Year Change Scores For All Patients

| Source | df | Target Symptoms | | Work Inadequacy | | Social Isolation | |
|---|---|---|---|---|---|---|---|
| | | M.S. | F | M.S. | F | M.S. | F |
| Treatments | 2 | 26.01 | 2.78 | 5.09 | 1.27 | .54 | .22 |
| Neuroticism | 1 | 2.50 | .27 | .79 | .20 | 3.33 | 1.33 |
| Sex | 1 | .07 | .01 | .81 | .20 | 2.76 | 1.10 |
| Treatments X neuroticism | 2 | .43 | .05 | 7.63 | 1.91 | .70 | .28 |
| Treatments X sex | 2 | 3.91 | .42 | 1.03 | .26 | .49 | .19 |
| Neuroticism X sex | 1 | 11.85 | 1.27 | 4.75 | 1.19 | 9.76 | 3.90[a] |
| Treatments X sex X neuroticism | 2 | .56 | .06 | 3.85 | .96 | 5.59 | 2.24 |
| Error | 78 | 9.35 | | 3.99 | | 2.50 | |
| Total | 89 | | | | | | |

[a] $p < .05$

provement at the four-month assessment did not continue treatment. Table 16 shows the mean improvement on target symptoms, work adjustment, and social isolation at four months for those who then received further treatment and for those who did not. There was some tendency for patients improving less to seek further treatment, particularly in the wait-list group, but this trend was not as clear or consistent for those patients who received psychotherapy or behavior therapy. The difference in improvement between "continuers" and "terminators" was statistically significant only for the social adjustment of psychotherapy patients. The difference in this case appeared to result from some worsening of continuers, rather than any marked improvement on the part of terminators. Amount of improvement at four months did appear to play some role in the patient's decision, but the amount of original improvement shown by the three no-further-treatment groups was essentially similar.

2. The group of terminators was made up both of patients who showed great improvement and those who became worse or showed no change, the latter having become discouraged from seeking further treatment. Thus, a mean improvement score, based on the average change shown by such a mixed group of terminators, might prove misleading and might not differ appreciably from the moderate change shown by continuers. In this case, however, the variance of the improvement scores should be higher for terminators than for continuers. Standard deviations of improvement scores are also shown in Table 16. While there was some tendency for the variance of terminators' scores to exceed those of continuers, such differences are slight and do not approach statistical significance.

3. The problems shown by continuers were initially more severe than those of terminators. While they might have shown equal improvement, continuers might still need treatment to a

TABLE 16. Patients Receiving Further Treatment Compared with Those Who Did Not: Self-Rating of Target Symptoms, Work, and Social Adjustment

| | | Behavior Therapy | | | Psychotherapy | | | Wait List | | | |
|---|---|---|---|---|---|---|---|---|---|---|---|
| | | Further Treatment | No Further Treatment | t | Further Treatment | No Further Treatment | t | Treatment | No Treatment | t | F |
| Target symptom | $\bar{x}$ | 1.64 | 1.25 | 1.439 | 1.22 | 1.44 | .556 | .37 | 1.07 | 2.654[a] | 1.889 |
| change | s | .66 | .69 | | .98 | .89 | | .62 | .64 | | |
| Work inadequacy | $\bar{x}$ | .77 | 1.71 | 1.521 | .53 | .40 | .322 | .28 | 1.52 | 1.742 | .286 |
| change | s | 1.47 | 1.58 | | .68 | 1.42 | | 1.32 | 1.92 | | |
| Social Isolation | $\bar{x}$ | .72 | .42 | .452 | -.32 | .68 | 2.195[a] | .89 | 1.02 | .251 | .413 |
| change | s | 1.46 | 1.81 | | .93 | 1.37 | | 1.17 | 1.31 | | |
| Initial target | $\bar{x}$ | 3.09 | 2.80 | 1.425 | 3.11 | 3.11 | 000 | 3.09 | 2.80 | 1.135 | 1.732 |
| symptom | s | .56 | .44 | | .42 | .54 | | .70 | .58 | | |
| Initial work | $\bar{x}$ | 3.78 | 4.83 | 1.422 | 3.81 | 3.07 | .982 | 3.12 | 3.97 | 1.210 | 4.509[a] |
| inadequacy | s | 1.82 | 1.84 | | 1.92 | 1.41 | | 1.75 | 1.67 | | |
| Initial social | $\bar{x}$ | 3.36 | 3.37 | .014 | 2.98 | 3.06 | .098 | 3.44 | 3.66 | .387 | .642 |
| isolation | s | 1.45 | .96 | | 2.07 | 1.53 | | 1.25 | 1.40 | | |
| Target symptom | $\bar{x}$ | 25.42 | 25.44 | .012 | 25.83 | 25.79 | .022 | 19.80 | 25.25 | 2.228[a] | .031 |
| improvement (self-rating) | s | 4.41 | 5.50 | | 3.48 | 5.36 | | 6.27 | 4.71 | | |
| Therapist | $\bar{x}$ | 5.60 | 6.57 | 1.851 | 5.55 | 6.21 | 1.506 | – | – | – | .489 |
| attraction | s | 1.20 | 1.50 | | .83 | 1.36 | | | | | |

[a] $p < .05$

greater extent. Comparisons of target symptom severity, work pathology, and social isolation scores at initial assessment (Table 16) do not support this view. However, psychotherapy terminators showed a lower initial level of work inadequacy than did other terminators.

4. The patient's own perception, rather than an observer's, might determine the decision whether to continue treatment or not. Table 16 shows the mean improvement on three target symptoms as rated by the patient. While there were no differences for either of the actively treated groups, wait-list patients who wished to start therapy did in fact perceive significantly less symptomatic improvement in themselves during the initial four-month period than those who decided not to begin treatment. Terminators in all three groups perceived a similar degree of improvement.

5. The patients might continue if the therapist liked them but discontinue if he did not. This was not so. The degree of attraction shown by the therapist did not differentiate the groups (Table 16).

6. Other demographic and personality characteristics might predispose toward termination. There were, however, no significant differences between continuers and terminators in age, intelligence, years of education, family size, income, marital status, or sex (Table 17). There was some tendency for a disproportionate number of females and first-born patients to seek further treatment.

7. There might be differences among assessors in the extent to which their patients sought further treatment. Approximately 41% of the patients seen by Assessor X, 40% of those seen by Assessor Y, and 60% of those seen by Assessor Z went on for further treatment. This nonsignificant difference might reflect either differences in assessors' attitudes about the value of further treatment, or the amounts of therapeutic support their own interviews provided.

TABLE 17. Patients Receiving Further Treatment Compared with Those Who Did Not: Demographic and Personality Characteristics

| | | Behavior Therapy | | | Psychotherapy | | | Wait List | | | |
|---|---|---|---|---|---|---|---|---|---|---|---|
| | | Further Treatment | No Further Treatment | t | Further Treatment | No Further Treatment | t | Treatment | No Treatment | t | F |
| Age | $\bar{x}$ | 24.87 | 24.57 | .120 | 21.00 | 24.22 | 1.822 | 21.68 | 24.42 | 2.732 | .010 |
| | s | 5.18 | 7.32 | | 2.31 | 6.47 | | 3.95 | 6.86 | | |
| I.Q. | $\bar{x}$ | 34.40 | 36.71 | .755 | 36.67 | 33.44 | 1.027 | 34.32 | 33.58 | .195 | .527 |
| (raw score) | s | 8.07 | 7.85 | | 5.69 | 9.92 | | 9.42 | 10.37 | | |
| Years education | $\bar{x}$ | 13.93 | 14.77 | 1.174 | 15.11 | 15.33 | .348 | 14.59 | 13.67 | 1.152 | 2.593 |
| | s | 1.91 | 1.72 | | 1.20 | 1.97 | | 2.21 | 1.97 | | |
| Number of | $\bar{x}$ | 1.47 | 2.92 | 1.478 | 1.67 | 2.00 | .333 | 2.15 | 2.15 | .006 | 1.450 |
| siblings | s | 1.15 | 3.25 | | 1.05 | 1.54 | | 2.31 | 1.51 | | |
| Income | $\bar{x}$ | 4.00 | 4.82 | .431 | 4.13 | 5.11 | .690 | 6.15 | 4.90 | .833 | .128 |
| | s | 3.27 | 5.27 | | 3.22 | 3.09 | | 3.80 | 3.65 | | |
| Sex, % female | | 67 | 54 | | 56 | 57 | | 78 | 50 | | |
| Married % | | 27 | 14 | | 11 | 27 | | 10 | 46 | | |
| First born % | | 67 | 46 | | 67 | 59 | | 45 | 31 | | |

8. There might be differences in attitudes toward further treatment between the therapists of the two persuasions. This proved to be the case. In fact, fewer psychotherapy than behavior therapy patients continued therapy. Paradoxically, the psychotherapists structured their therapy within a four-month framework and, having told the patients they would see them for only four months, were reluctant to extend it. However, those who continued in psychotherapy tended to receive more therapy than those who persevered with behavior therapy. In part this was probably a matter of style. Behavior therapists are more prone to have occasional "topping up" sessions with patients than psychotherapists. The latter, once embarked on continuing therapy, are more inclined to make it a regular occurrence.

Thus, the decision to continue or forgo further treatment appeared to be mainly determined by the particular treatment group and assessor seen by the patient. The characteristics of the patient and the amount of improvement were of lesser importance. Since there were no marked differences among the subgroups of terminators, and since they appeared reasonably representative of their whole treatment groups, we decided to compare the three treatments by examining improvement shown by those patients in each group who received no treatment after the initial four-month period. Thus we compared fourteen behavior therapy, twenty-one psychotherapy, and eleven wait-list patients.

Mean scores for the three subgroups at initial, four-month, and one-year assessments are shown for the three measures in Figures 15, 16, and 17. All three groups maintained their original improvement on target symptoms and remained significantly improved over their initial status at one year. The amount of improvement shown was similar for all three groups, as there were no significant between-group differences (Table 18).

Figure 15

Target Symptom Severity:
Mean Ratings of Patients Who Received No Treatment
after Four Months

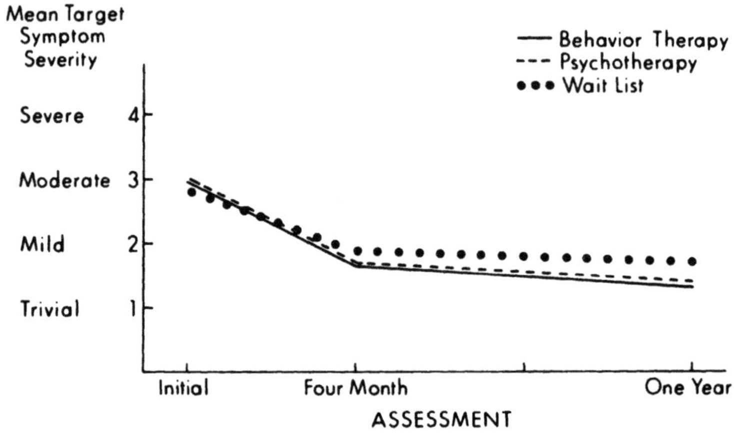


Figure 16

Work Inadequacy:
Assessor SSIAM Ratings of Patients Who Received No Treatment
after Four Months

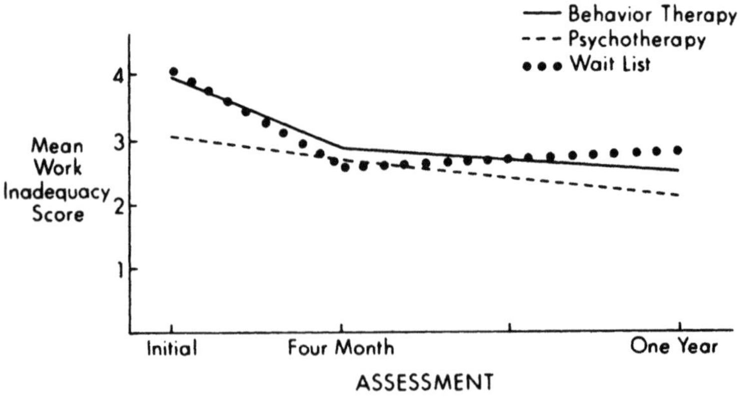

Figure 17

Social Isolation:
Assessor SSIAM Ratings of Patients Who Received No Treatment after Four Months

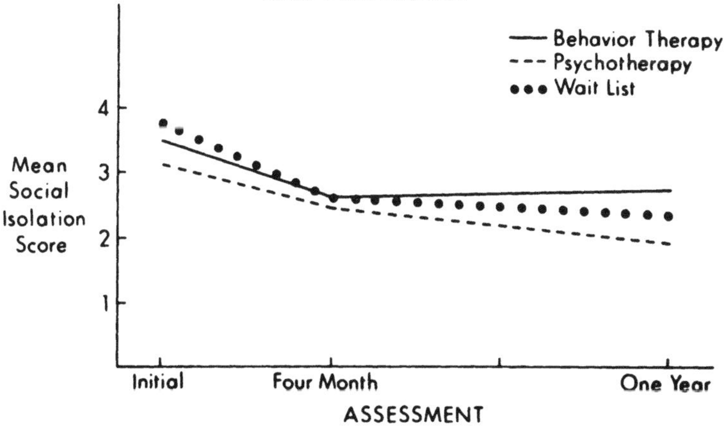


A similar pattern was shown for work and social pathology, although improvement was somewhat less consistent. Improvement at one year was "marginally" significant for wait-list patients on work, and for both behavior therapy and wait-list patients on social adjustment. Again, however, there were no significant group differences in amount of improvement shown (Table 18).

## CASE ILLUSTRATIONS

Evelyn Ashley, the tense college senior, was still doing well at her one-year assessment. She had received no further psychotherapy after four months. She had been happily married for several months now, and her tension, feelings of inadequacy, and lifelong tendency to escape into fantasy were all completely recovered. Her relationship with her mother had improved, and she felt much more self-confident in social situations. Her husband (who had been her informant before their marriage as well) told the research

TABLE 18. Changes from Initial to One-Year Assessment in Patients Receiving No Further Treatment

| | Behavior Therapy | | Psycho-therapy | | Wait List | | |
|---|---|---|---|---|---|---|---|
| | d | t | d | t | d | t | F |
| Target symptoms | 4.714 | $6.422^{a}$ | 4.905 | $6.907^{a}$ | 3.143 | $3.640^{a}$ | 1.487 |
| Work inadequacy | 1.446 | $2.231^{b}$ | .929 | $2.526^{b}$ | 1.250 | $1.974^{c}$ | .286 |
| Social isolation | .829 | $1.991^{c}$ | 1.229 | $4.136^{a}$ | 1.400 | $2.097^{c}$ | .413 |

$^{a}p < .001$
$^{b}p < .05$
$^{c}p < .05$ (one-tailed)

assistant that she seemed more light-hearted and things didn't bother her as much.

After her four-month assessment Marie Sutton, the opera singer, had received a few additional sessions of psychotherapy and was still doing extremely well. Her singing was going superbly, and she was now tense for one day, instead of two or three weeks, before each performance. Never again had she had the feeling that she was about to pass out; her tension was reduced still further and her concentration was still good.

Emma Hubbard had received six months of psychotherapy from a senior resident by the time of her one-year assessment. She was still fat but she liked her therapist and felt she was gaining insight into her feelings and reactions. Apart from a reduction in nervousness there was little objective change. She had gained ten pounds, was still not dating, and perhaps felt slightly less self-conscious. She was globally rated as unchanged, but the assessor felt she was a difficult case for any form of brief therapy, and that the next year might bring real improvment. (Six months later she had lost forty pounds and was making corresponding social gains.)

At the one-year reassessment, Tom Morton had consolidated his earlier gains with no further behavior therapy. He was enrolled in medical school, doing extremely well, and enjoying it. His loneliness, lack of values, and need to impress people were still much improved, and the assessor noticed that Tom seemed to have less need to make a favorable impression on him. He had broken off with his previous girlfriend and was now enjoying sex more. Tom's mother agreed that he had calmed down considerably and was much more relaxed. His therapist was now treating Tom's parents, and "we are a happier family". Overall Tom was rated very much improved.

Raymond Simpson's symptoms—eye twitching, great social anxiety, depression, difficulty working, compulsive eating—were still unchanged at the one-year reassessment. His complexion was somewhat improved but he had become noticeably overweight. His grades were barely passing, he had dropped one major course because of inability to concentrate, and he had developed insomnia. He expressed in strong terms his feeling that everybody connected with the study was using him. The entire experience had been impersonal, "like assembly-line therapy," and had disenchanted if not actually harmed him. He still wanted therapy, but on a longer-term basis and certainly not with his original psychotherapist. His assessor made arrangements for him to see another experienced therapist.

Veneta Williams, the black social worker, had two additional sessions of psychotherapy after her four-month assessment. At one year, her loneliness and lack of friends were still problems, but her target symptoms were all completely recovered. Her brother felt she had improved considerably since the four-month assessment, and said she had relaxed, was warmer, was enjoying her work more, and was getting along better with her family.

Norman Rollins, the tense government clerk, had no further psychotherapy after four months, but he was still happy at his one-year assessment. He seemed relaxed, his pinched look had not returned, and he carried himself more erectly, appearing taller than he had a year before. His social anxiety, fears for his wife and child, and other target symptoms were all very much better or completely recovered. He had graduated from night college and had been given a fellowship to social work school, where he was doing well academically and also getting along well with people. He felt he was growing more independent, assertive, and strong, and he could tolerate criticism much better than previously. He no longer had long arguments with his wife. He and the assessor both felt that he was vastly improved. His wife again told the research assistant that he had not changed, and that any change was due to altered circumstances, not to therapy. Yet she mentioned a number of the same specific improvements her husband had emphasized.

Louise Shaw, the fearful housewife, had no behavior therapy after the four-month interview, and at one year she had relapsed almost to her original state, with severe fear of a urinary accident and of going out. This exacerbation was precipitated by a quarrel between her and her sister about who should support their aging father, which had awakened all her early parental conflicts. It was suggested that she get more therapy. But although she had liked her therapist and felt he had helped her, she now despaired of any therapy's offering her permanent help. Her target symptoms were rated as slightly better than at the original interview. Her husband told the research assistant that although she forced herself to go places this was still very difficult for her.

Mary Teresa Moore had married and was happily pregnant at the time of her one-year assessment. She was prettier, talked more spontaneously, and had none of the nervous-rat appearance of her initial interview. Her target symptoms were all completely recovered, and she had no worries about harming her children, or anything else. She still had some guilt feelings related to sex but generally enjoyed her sex life, and it seemed that this would improve gradually with time. The assessor felt that therapy played an important role in her recovery. The marriage certainly helped, but she indicated that therapy had helped her make up her mind to go through with the marriage, and had helped make her a better wife. "She is very happy in her marriage and feels that life is idyllic."

## FOURTH ASSESSMENT

About two years after the initial assessment, 61 patients returned for a final follow-up interview with the research assistant, and shortly thereafter 48 patients took the MMPI again. Six patients had refused to return for a final assessment. The remainder could not be located, many having moved from the city. At this time the great majority of patients in all groups had increased or maintained significant improvement, both on symptomatic and adjustment measures and on the MMPI scales. However, this proved to be a biased sample. The psychotherapy patients who returned for this follow-up had improved significantly more *in the first year* than had the behavior therapy patients who returned for it. The behavior therapy and wait list patients who returned for follow-up were apparently representative of their whole groups. Because of this bias we could not properly compare the groups.

Only seven of these patients had had any substantial amount of therapy since their one-year assessment, yet there were few relapses and many had continued to improve. This is clear evidence that the earlier significant improvement was neither transitory nor maintained only by continued supportive therapy, and suggests that lasting change can be produced by competent, experienced therapists.

This evidence is not diminished by the continued improvement of the wait-list group. By final follow-up the latter had received as much therapy as the treated groups and was no longer a control group. Thus, the fact that control patients ultimately reached the same level of adjustment as the treated patients may only reflect that by this time, "control" patients were treated patients. It is not evidence for Frank's [1] view that therapy primarily accelerates spontaneous change rather than producing unique change.

## PATIENT RATINGS OF OUTCOME

At one year, group differences in patient ratings of improvement tended to disappear in the same way as assessor ratings. Figures 18 and 19 show the mean group ratings of improvement, and Tables 19, 20, 21, and 22 show analyses of variance, for all patients and for those subgroups who received no further treatment after four months. While patients in both original active treatment groups tended to consider themselves more improved in all areas, none of the between-group differences approached statistical significance. The lack of more pronounced differences at one year does not appear to result from deterioration among treated groups. These patients felt they had, on the average, maintained or augmented their earlier gains. It was rather the wait-list patients, both those

Figure 18

Improvement at One Year for All Patients: Rated by Patients

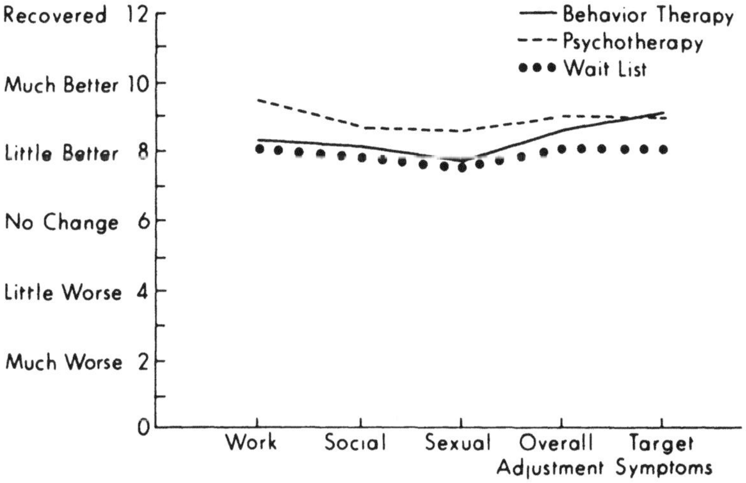


who received treatment and those who did not, who felt they had improved more between four months and one year.

## CONCLUSIONS

In this study behavior therapy was at least as effective, and perhaps more so, than psychoanalytically oriented psychotherapy in treating patients with typical mixed neuroses. There was little difference between the two active treatments in amount of improvement. It would be tempting to argue that behavior therapy was somewhat more effective than psychotherapy. At four months, behavior therapy patients had significantly improved on all three measures, while psychotherapy patients had not improved on social adjustment. At one year, patients who were originally treated by behavior therapy, but not those originally treated by psychotherapy,

Figure 19

Improvement at One Year for Patients
Who Received No Treatment after Four Months:
Rated by Patients

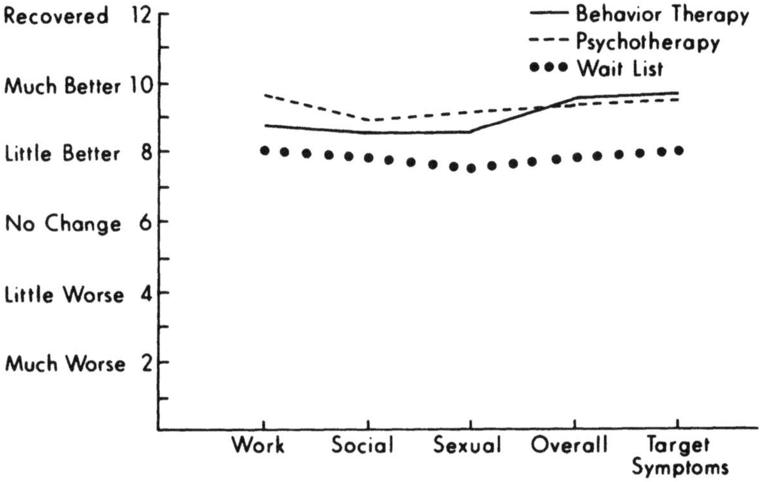


TABLE 19. Target Symptom Severity and Overall Adjustment at One Year: Analyses of Variance of Comparative Ratings by Patients

| | Target Symptoms | | | Overall Adjustment | | |
|---|---|---|---|---|---|---|
| Source | df | M.S. | F | df | M.S. | F |
| Treatments | 2 | 99.99 | 2.134 | 2 | 7.30 | 1.152 |
| Within groups | 87 | 46.86 | | 90 | 6.34 | |
| Total | 89 | | | 92 | | |

showed greater improvement than wait-list patients in reduction of severity of target symptoms.

Such a conclusion is tempered by the finding of no significant difference between the two groups in amount of improvement in social adjustment at four months. Also the com-

TABLE 20. Work, Social, and Sexual Adjustment at One Year: Analyses of Variance of Comparative Ratings by Patients

| Source | Work Adjustment | | | Social Adjustment | | | Sexual Adjustment | | |
|---|---|---|---|---|---|---|---|---|---|
| | df | M.S. | F | df | M.S. | F | df | M.S. | F |
| Treatments | 2 | 14.92 | 2.567 | 2 | 5.49 | .868 | 2 | 10.04 | 1.582 |
| Within groups | 86 | 5.81 | | 90 | 6.32 | | 89 | 6.35 | |
| Total | 88 | | | 92 | | | 91 | | |

TABLE 21. Target Symptom Severity and Overall Adjustment at One Year for Patients Who Received No Further Treatment: Analyses of Variance of Comparative Ratings by Patients

| | Target Symptoms | | | Overall Adjustment | | |
|---|---|---|---|---|---|---|
| Source | df | M.S. | F | df | M.S. | F |
| Treatments | 2 | 94.67 | 1.660 | 2 | 11.06 | 1.686 |
| Within groups | 41 | 57.03 | | 42 | 6.56 | |
| Total | 43 | | | 44 | | |

parison of the two full groups at one year was confounded by different amounts of treatment after four months. Several behavior therapy patients in fact received subsequent psychotherapy.

Previous comparative studies have tended to show behavior therapy as more effective than traditional therapy, either in terms of greater or more rapid improvement. However, the procedure of the present study differed from these previous ones in a number of significant ways.

*All therapists were well qualified*, experienced practitioners, in contrast to the psychiatric residents, graduate students in psychology, and other relatively inexperienced therapists used in several other studies. Since it is recognized that competence in analytically oriented therapy requires more training and experience than is required for some behavioral techniques, behavior therapy may have had a built-in advantage in previous studies.

*Therapists in this study were not limited in techniques used.* Comparative studies with behavior therapy have frequently used only systematic desensitization. Since behavior therapy is more than systematic desensitization, sometimes much more,[2] such studies are more properly a test of the technique of sys-

TABLE 22. Work, Social, and Sexual Adjustment at One Year for Patients Who Received No Further Treatment: Analyses of Variance of Comparative Ratings by Patients

| Source | Work Adjustment | | | Social Adjustment | | | Sexual Adjustment | | |
|---|---|---|---|---|---|---|---|---|---|
| | df | M.S. | F | df | M.S. | F | df | M.S. | F |
| Treatments | 2 | 10.22 | 1.357 | 2 | 4.27 | .561 | 2 | 9.61 | 1.421 |
| Within groups | 41 | 7.53 | | 43 | 7.61 | | 42 | 6.76 | |
| Total | 43 | | | 45 | | | 44 | | |

tematic desensitization than behavior therapy in the broad sense.

*Our subjects were real patients suffering from a variety of disorders.* Results of analogue studies involving student volunteers rather than real patients, while providing useful information, may not necessarily be generalized directly to patient populations.

*Experienced clinical observers evaluated therapeutic gains.* Unlike therapist raters, they were not involved in the treatments and could remain open-minded about possible outcomes. There was, in fact, no evidence of bias in favor of one therapy by any of the assessors.

These major procedural differences between the present study and previous ones may account for differences in outcome.

Behavior therapy and psychotherapy were clearly more effective than the minimal contact treatment only in producing greater symptomatic relief at the end of the initial treatment period. The lack of more pronounced differences between active treatment groups and the wait list appeared to result from the high rate of improvement shown by minimal contact patients.

Both active treatments were highly effective. Of the patients who had received treatment only during the first four months, 90% were improved on target symptoms, 70% on work, and 75% on social adjustment at one year.

Striking was the absence of the deterioration so often found even at the hands of experienced therapists. Only two patients (one wait list and one psychotherapy) were considered worse by the assessor on overall adjustment. This also emphasizes the therapeutic aspects of the wait list. In fact, the improvement shown by the wait-list patients may have resulted from a number of factors. Because of the minimal contact treatment given these patients, the wait list cannot be regarded as a passive control group. A number of therapeutic factors were operative.

1. Wait-list patients made an active commitment to improvement. Not only did they seek help on their own initiative, but publicly declared this by bringing a friend or relative. They also invested considerable time and psychic energy in the assessment procedures. Patients at the initial interview spent approximately one-half hour giving socioeconomic and other information, two and one-half hours with the assessing psychiatrist, one and one-half hours in testing for another study, and then took home several lengthy questionnaires including the MMPI and CPI to complete. As Goldstein has demonstrated, such public and personal commitment to recovery can have a pronounced effect.[3]

2. The diagnostic interview itself could be considered a therapeutic tool. Patients had the opportunity to discuss their problems in depth with an experienced, sympathetic psychiatrist. Several found this extremely helpful. In addition, the assessor's assurance that therapy would be beneficial and that a therapist would be assigned as soon as possible aroused hope and the expectation of improvement.

3. Patients were given a card bearing the name and telephone number of the assessor and of the Psychiatry Department Crisis Center. They were told to call in the event of any crisis or emergency. The periodic telephone calls the research assistant made to inquire about the patient's health reinforced the impression that there was professional help available and that people cared about him.

# 6 Differences Between Behavior Therapy and Psychotherapy

This chapter describes the differences between behavior therapy and analytically oriented psychotherapy as actually practiced by therapists in the study. Therapists were not restricted to specific techniques such as desensitization or assertive training. Within the broad framework of behavior therapy or of insight therapy they were free to use whatever procedure they felt would most benefit the patient. However, before any therapy began, all therapists endorsed a list of stipulative definitions defining characteristics of the two treatments and providing a crude framework or set of ground rules. These can be found in Appendix 3.

However, these definitions merely set limits of allowable techniques and do not define what therapists actually did in treatment. Without empirical measures of actual therapy behavior, it could be argued that we compared therapists who said they were doing behavior therapy and therapists who said they were doing analytically oriented psychotherapy. Consequently, independent measures of therapist behavior were taken. These measures allowed the two therapies to be compared in a number of dimensions: first, the formal characteristics of the patient-therapist interaction; second, the nature of the patient-therapist relationship; and third, the specific clinical techniques used in treatment.

Formal characteristics of patient-therapist interaction were compared by using routinely-made tape recordings of the fifth interviews between patient and therapist. Due to technical difficulties, only fifty of these could be subsequently transcribed (twenty-eight from behavior therapy and twenty-two from psychotherapy). From these tapes and transcripts we compared behavior therapists and analytically oriented psychotherapists with respect to patient-therapist interaction patterns. These interviews appeared representative of the treatments when compared with spot checks of the third and tenth interviews.

## TRUAX THERAPIST VARIABLES

Truax and his associates have demonstrated the potent effect on outcome of treatment of such therapist variables as self-congruence, accurate empathy, depth of interpersonal contact, and unconditional positive regard.[1] These measures, originally devised to test assumptions of Rogerian nondirective counseling, may describe basic parameters of the interaction between therapist and patient. They probably represent valid dimensions of therapist behavior in general.

Four four-minute samples were selected from tape recordings of the fifth interview. We tried to obtain a representative sample of the verbal interaction in each quarter of the interview. Within each quarter, sample selection was not entirely random. In a few cases, most often in behavior therapy, a randomly selected sample contained little patient verbalization because some particular technique (e.g., desensitization) was being used by the therapist, and in these cases another more representative sample was selected.

Samples were independently scored, according to Truax's criteria, by two raters who had previous experience with his scoring system. There was an acceptable degree of interrater agreement. Correlations between the two independent ratings ranged from .58 to .74. Discrepancies between raters were settled by taking the mean value of the two ratings. A single index for each variable for each interview was taken by averaging across samples from each of the four quarters.

The graphic representation of the differences between behavior therapists and psychotherapists can be understood as follows. We calculated means and standard deviations for each treatment group for each variable. These are plotted in the form of bar graphs, with the standard deviation for each group represented by the height of the bar and the mean value for that group represented by a solid line through the middle of the bar. Thus in Figure 20, the first shaded bar shows the ratings of the 28 behavior therapy samples for Depth of Inter-Personal Contact. The white bar shows the values for the 22 psychotherapy samples. The mean value for the behavior therapy group is 4.08 (represented by the horizontal line) with a standard deviation of .347 (plotted from 3.91 to 4.25 equidistant above and below the mean). The heavy line between the two bars represents the difference between the two means which would be required for statistical significance at the .05 level for a two-tailed *t* test for the N and size of the standard deviations.

Thus, if the heavy line between the two bars overlaps the horizontal lines representing the mean values, there is no statistically significant difference between the behavior therapy and psychotherapy groups. If the line does not overlap the means, the groups differ significantly at the .05 level of confidence. In the first case, depth of interpersonal contact, the heavy line does not overlap the means because behavior therapists showed a significantly higher level of interpersonal contact than did psychotherapists.

In addition, behavior therapists showed a significantly

Figure 20

Truax Variables for Behavior Therapists and Psychotherapists During Fifth Interview

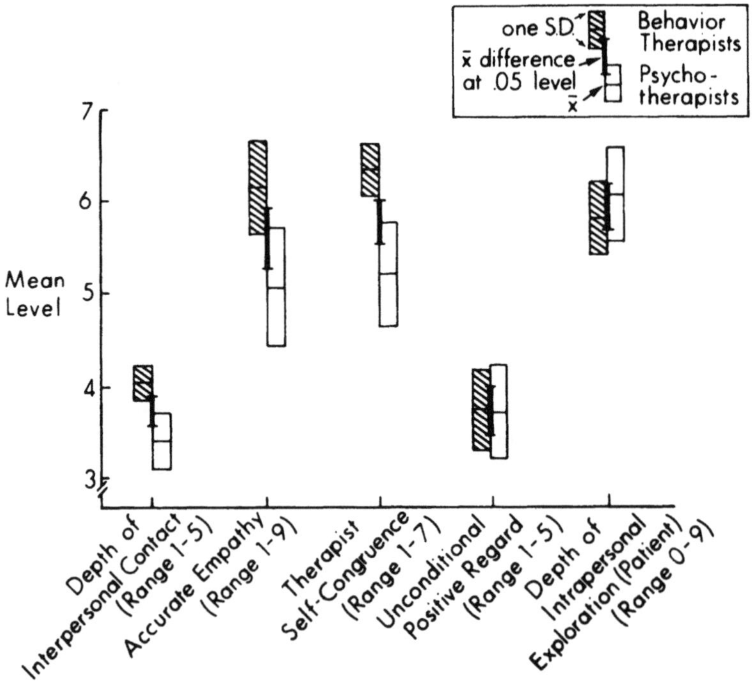


higher level of Accurate Empathy and of Therapist Self-Congruence than did psychotherapists. Both showed an equal degree of warmth or unconditional positive regard toward the patient. This is somewhat surprising in view of the fact that behavior therapy has been at times characterized as a rather impersonal process with little regard for the patient as a human being in contrast to the close empathic relationship of psychotherapy. However, both groups of therapists showed high levels of these variables.

On the interpersonal contact scale, behavior therapists were functioning at about stage four in intensity and intimacy, which indicates they were "concernedly attentive" to the patient, while the psychotherapists were between stages three and four. (Stage three is "attentive but not engrossed".) On the accurate empathy scale behavior therapists were functioning at a level "recognizing most of the client's present feelings, including those which are not readily apparent, although they may misjudge the intensity of some of the veiled ones". Psychotherapists, at the next lowest stage, "gave an accurate response to the obvious feelings and had an awareness at least of the more hidden ones".

Behavior therapists were operating at the second highest stage in therapist self-congruence scales, indicating that "they displayed genuine feeling, and meant what they said, although they did not say all they could". Psychotherapists, at least one stage lower, "expressed genuine feeling, although it might be muted or restrained". Both groups showed a similar degree of unconditional positive regard. There was considerable warmth or regard shown but it was not unconditional. For example, the therapist "communicated a desire for improvement and for being liked himself".

Perhaps more surprising than the differences in therapist characteristics was the lack of difference in depth of patient intrapersonal exploration. This variable describes the extent to which the patient discusses his problems on a meaningful rather than a superficial level. It might have been expected that patients in psychotherapy would have discussed their problems on a deeper level than would patients of behavior therapists, but again, this was not so.

## LENNARD AND BERNSTEIN CATEGORIES

Another measure of the interaction between patient and therapist is the degree of control the therapist exerts over the interaction. At one extreme, such as in client-centered counseling, the therapist exerts little control over the patient's verbalization. The responsibility for maintaining conversation is placed almost entirely on the patient. By contrast, in a more highly structured diagnostic interview, the onus is on the therapist or interviewer to elicit the kinds of information he wants from the interviewee or patient. This dimension is relevant to understanding differences between behavior therapy and psychotherapy as well. In analytically oriented psychotherapy the focus of attention is on the patient's verbalization and free association. The initiative for interaction is basically the patient's responsibility. It might be expected, therefore, that psychotherapists would exert less control over the content of the interaction and allow patients to talk about a greater variety of topics at their own discretion than would behavior therapists.

Lennard and Bernstein designed a scale to measure the degree of therapist control over the content of the interaction.[2] They described their scale as follows:

> Any idea (proposition) expressed by a therapist may be regarded as a message sent to the patient by the therapist. Such propositions differ in the degree to which the information provides a basis for limiting the range or array of possible responses. For example, the therapist statement, 'just start by saying anything that occurs to you,' has the lowest specific informational stimulus value, because it does not limit the patient's response to any specific subject matter or proposition. It may therefore be said to be nondirective or unstructured. On the other hand, the question 'how old are your sisters?' has a high information stimulus value because it provides information that can be used to set limits on a range of possible alternatives from which the patient may select his reply. It

> therefore may be said to be highly directive or structured. To adapt these notions to the study of informational structure of therapist verbal output during psychotherapy, a set of eight categories was devised to roughly quantify the amount of structure or information contained in each therapist message. The amount of information contained in any therapist proposition is defined as its 'informational stimulus value.' This corresponds to the extent to which it tends to place limits upon the array of verbal responses from which the patient may choose or reply.

The same interview samples used for the Truax ratings were also used for the Lennard and Bernstein Therapist Informational Specificity Scale. Figure 21 shows the frequency of each category of statements for behavior therapists and psychotherapists.

While the differences between categories do not represent an equal interval scale, higher numbered categories reflect greater degree of informational specificity, and thus greater control over the topic of discussion, than do the lower categories. The categories are described in some detail in Appendix 5.

These ratings indicated that behavior therapists tended to control the content of conversation more than psychotherapists. Psychotherapists used more statements that encourage the patient to carry on with, or else follow directly from, whatever topic the patient has raised (categories 1, 2, 3 in Figure 21). Behavior therapists, on the other hand, used more statements that introduce new topics or seek new information. Put another way, the topic discussed tends to be initiated by the patient in psychotherapy and by the therapist in behavior therapy.

## SPEECH PATTERNS

A third variable that describes the relationship between patient and therapist is the pattern of speech and silence in the

Figure 21

Therapist Informational Specificity Ratings During Fifth Interview

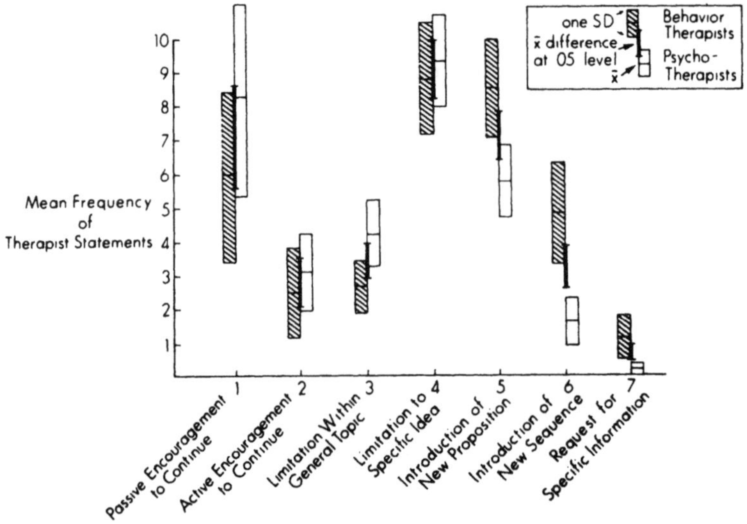


interview. Analysis of these nonlexical speech characteristics, while providing no information on the content of the conversation, defines the basic form of the interaction in the therapeutic dyad. Tapes of the fifth interview were timed while following a transcript of the interview. In portions of a few interviews, most often in behavior therapy, the therapist used some technique that disrupted the usual interaction. These periods were omitted from the analyses.

Figure 22 shows the means and standard deviations of therapist and patient total speech time, total pause time and "floor time". Total speech time refers to the amount of time that each participant spends talking. There were clear differences here. Behavior therapists spent roughly twice as much time talking as psychotherapists. The pattern was reversed for patient total speech time, because patients in psychotherapy spent

Figure 22

Therapist and Patient Speech and Pause Times

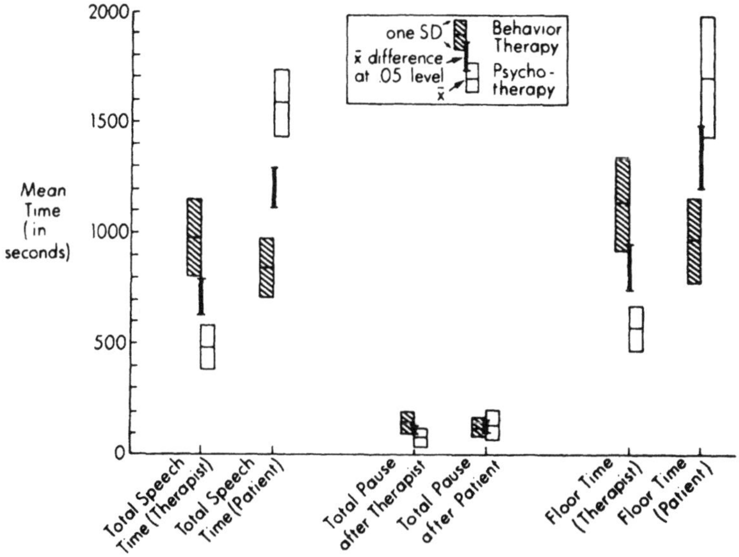


about twice as much time talking as did patients in behavior therapy. In behavior therapy there was a reasonably close match in the total amount of time spent in speech by the therapist and by the patient. In psychotherapy, however, the patient spent roughly three times as much time in speech as did the therapist.

The total pause time refers to the sum of the accumulated pause times after the therapist finishes a statement before the patient responds, or until the therapist begins to speak again. As can be seen, there was a statistically significant intergroup difference in total pause time following therapist speech but not following patient speech.

The third variable in Figure 22, floor time, refers to the total length of time the conversation is controlled by each participant. Floor time is simply the sum of the total speech time plus the total pause time after that individual's speech. The pattern here was similar to the pattern for total speech time; behavior therapists held the floor roughly twice as much as psychotherapists, while the reverse was true for patients in either treatment.

The number of therapist and patient speech units and number of interruptions are shown in Figure 23. While there was some tendency for both behavior therapists and their patients to speak more often in the therapeutic hour than psy-

Figure 23

Therapist and Patient Speech Units and Interruptions

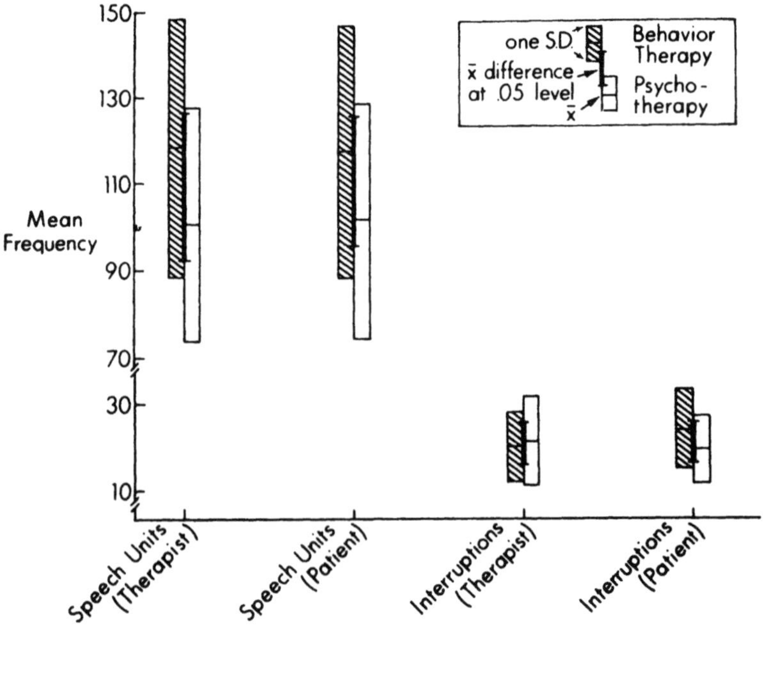

chotherapists and their patients, there was considerable overlap between the two groups and these differences did not approach statistical significance. There were no group differences in number of interruptions either by the therapist or the patient.

Average speech durations and average reaction times of therapists and patients are presented in Figure 24. Mean speech duration represents the average time taken to express a complete thought and includes time taken for brief pauses or disfluencies during the expression of a statement. This definition is similar to the one proposed by Matarazzo.[3]

Figure 24

Therapist and Patient Speech Durations and Reaction Times

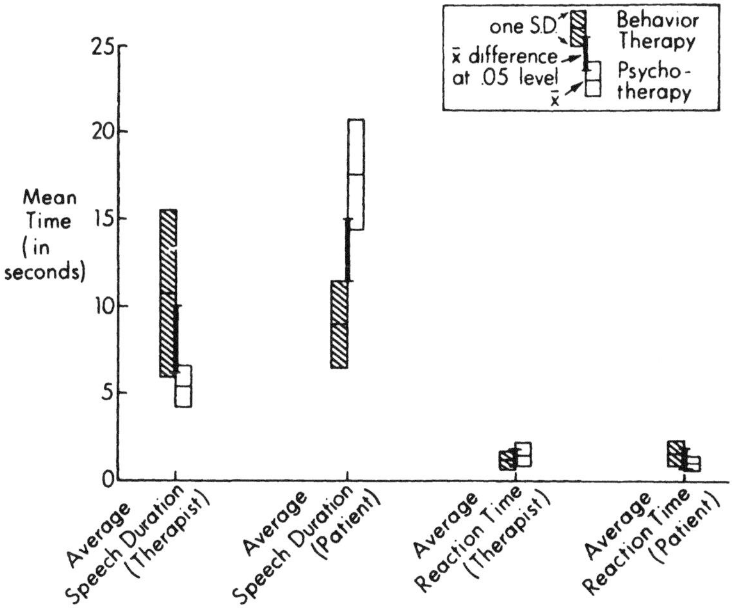

Behavior therapists' average speech durations were nearly twice as long as those of psychotherapists. Thus the difference between treatments in total therapist speech time resulted from longer rather than more frequent speech units by behavior therapists. Behavior therapists varied somewhat in their speech pattern. While the speech durations of psychotherapists tended to be quite similar, the senior behavior therapist spoke more frequently in short utterances while the second tended to give less frequent but longer statements.

The speech durations of patients in psychotherapy were roughly twice as long as those of patients in behavior therapy. As with therapist speech time, the greater total speech time by psychotherapy patients resulted from longer and not more frequent speech units.

There were no differences between therapists in how quickly they reacted to patients' verbalizations (average reaction times). Both groups responded quickly, with little variation. There was some tendency for behavior therapy patients to respond more slowly to their therapists than psychotherapy patients did.

The overall pattern of speech in the interview was quite different for behavior therapy and analytically oriented psychotherapy. Behavior therapists were much more active and tended to dominate the conversation to a greater extent than psychotherapists. Because their verbalizations were longer than those of psychotherapists, they took up a much higher proportion of the therapeutic hour with their speech. Indeed, they took as much time as their patients. Psychotherapists appeared to play a much more passive role, in the sense that they devoted more time to patient verbalization.

## TEMPLE CONTENT CATEGORIES

The Lennard and Bernstein ratings indicate how much the therapist controls the content of the conversation, but provide no information about the content itself or the manner in which the conversation is controlled. We decided to include a measure of the content of the therapist's part of the interaction. Our content categories derive basically from the Bales Interaction Scale, but were modified to test differences between the activity of behavior therapists and psychotherapists. More specifically, we suspected that behavior therapists might more frequently ask for information from the patient, give more items of specific information, be more directive in the sense of giving specific instructions, and also be more directly approving of their patients than psychotherapists. Psychotherapists, on the other hand, might give more nondirective statements and more statements designed to clarify and interpret the patients' psychological problems.

We developed a rating scale with the following categories:

1. Asking for information. This category includes statements designed to seek new information from the patient. It excludes questions that are intended to clarify rather than seek information. Statements such as "tell me" would be included here and not treated as a directive statement. ("When did your father die?")

2. Giving information. This category refers primarily to neutral information and excludes information designed to aid the patient in interpreting his own individual psychological problem. ("The bathroom's at the end of the hall.")

3. Clarification and interpretation. This category includes statements designed to clarify and interpret to the patient the causality of certain things, often (although not necessarily) along the theoretical model of the therapist. This includes the giving of psychological information that is directly related to the patient's individual problem. ("So it's mostly domineering women who make you pick your scalp.")

4. Nondirective statements. These include indirect indications of approval, such as reassurance and indications of

understanding, also statements which do not specifically ask for or give information. ("Mm-hmm.")

5. Directive statements. These imply imperatives such as "do this." ("Keep a detailed record of everything you eat next week.")

6. Approval. This includes direct approval given to the patient for his behavior or statements. ("I'm glad you did that.")

7. Disapproval. This includes direct expressions of disapproval of the patient's statements or behavior. ("I don't think you should do that.")

Transcripts of the fifth interview between patient and therapist were rated by two research assistants. Each counted the number of therapist statements that fell into each of the seven categories. Their ratings were highly reliable, ranging from .83 for category 3 to .97 for category 1. Any disagreements in ratings were settled by taking the mean of the two ratings for that category in that interview.

The frequency of the seven kinds of statements for behavior therapists and psychotherapists are shown in Figure 25. Those most used were information-seeking, interpretation, and nondirective. Direct expressions of approval or disapproval were given only rarely. The only group differences that reached statistical significance were in the categories of information-giving and directiveness. Behavior therapists made more statements providing information to the patient. This difference appeared to result from the greater readiness of behavior therapists to respond to direct questions by patients. Psychotherapists tended to reflect the patient's direct and indirect questions, whereas behavior therapists tended to answer these directly. Again it should be pointed out that items in this category do not refer to information directly related to the interpretation of the patient's problem.

There were no differences between therapists in the extent

Figure 25

Frequency of Therapist Statements in Each Content Category During Fifth Interview

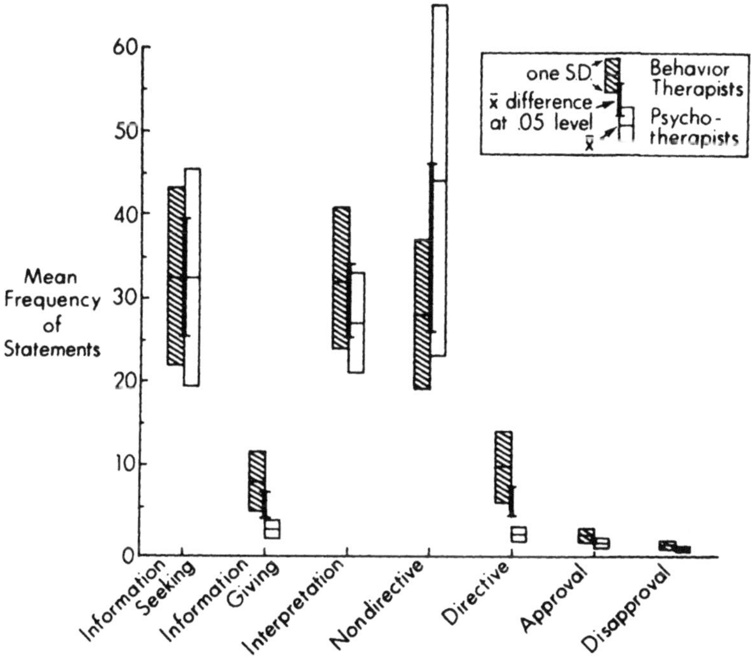


to which they used statements interpreting and clarifying the patient's problem. Such interpretation was broadly defined and not necessarily restricted to the relationship between the patient's feelings for the therapist and those toward his parents in childhood. Thus, the measure was not comparable to Malan's "transference-parent link".[4] Behavior therapists also used more statements prescribing certain courses of action for the patient to carry out. This is in keeping with the conception of the behavior therapist as a teacher who instructs the patient in more adaptive patterns of behavior. Thus more explicit instructions for action were given.

## THERAPIST ATTITUDE TOWARD THE PATIENT

At the end of four months' therapy, therapists rated each patient on a ten-item rating scale. The questions were designed to assess the quality of the therapeutic relationship from the therapist's point of view. They fall into three groups: (I) to measure the therapist's attraction toward the patient, (II) to measure the suitability of the patient for the therapist's treatment, and (III) to measure the patient's attitude toward the therapist.

*Group I.*

1. How did you feel toward this patient? (Disliked very much = 0; liked very much = 10)
3. How often did you feel uncomfortable? (At some time in every session = 0; never in any session = 10)
9. How interesting did you find the patient? (Extremely dull = 0; unusually interesting = 10)

*Group II.*

2. How suitable was this patient for your treatment? (Impossible = 0; excellent = 10)
7. How well did the patient understand your therapy? (Not at all = 0; completely = 10)
10. How much does this patient resemble or differ from your usual patients? (Most unusual = 0; very typical = 10)

*Group III.*

4. How did the patient feel about you? (Strongly disapproving = 0; strongly approving = 10)
5. How cooperative was the patient? (Extremely uncooperative = 0; extremely cooperative = 10)

6. How good a therapist did the patient think you were? (Extremely poor = 0; outstandingly good = 10)
8. How often did the patient criticize you? (A large part of every session = 0; not at all = 10)

Means and standard deviations of therapist ratings are shown for both kinds of therapists in Figure 26. There were no differences between them on any of the items reflecting attraction for the patient (1, 3, or 9). All therapists showed, on the average, a positive attitude toward the patient in terms of liking him, feeling comfortable with him, and finding him an interesting patient.

Psychotherapists felt that, on the average, their patients were less suitable for their treatment than did behavior therapists. The mean rating of psychotherapists was slightly below

Figure 26

Therapist Attitude Toward the Patient

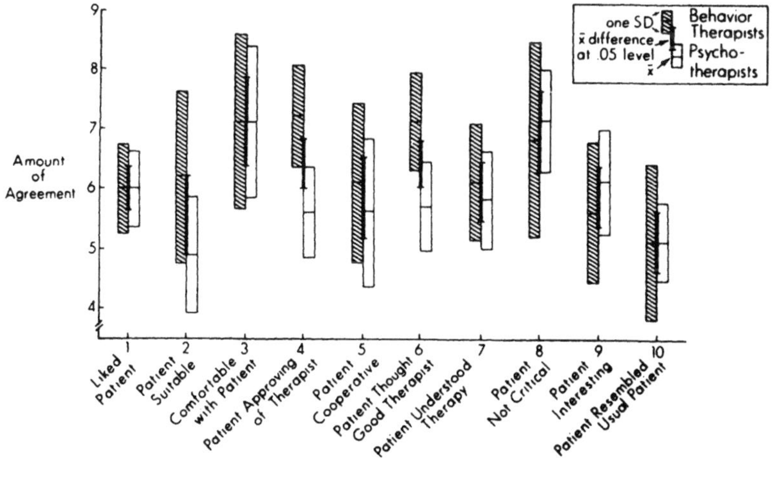

the midpoint of the scale, indicating that their patients tended to be rated toward the "impossible" rather than the "excellent" end of the scale as regards suitability for treatment. Differences here were also related to the experience level of the therapist. The senior therapists in both behavior therapy and psychotherapy considered their patients suitable while junior therapists of both disciplines felt patients were less than suitable. This tendency was more pronounced in the psychotherapy group and seems responsible for the overall difference evident in item (2). Similarly, while there were no overall between-therapy differences, there was a clear tendency for less experienced therapists of both kinds to perceive their patients as less similar to their usual patients, and showing less understanding of their treatment. This would suggest that senior therapists, because of their greater experience in dealing with a variety of patients, could assimilate such patients into their therapeutic framework better than junior therapists.

Behavior therapists felt that their patients perceived them as better therapists (6) and were more approving of them (4) than did psychotherapists. There were no such differences in degree of patient cooperation or amount of criticism received from the patient. All therapists felt, on the average, that patients perceived them as good therapists, approved of them, cooperated, and gave relatively little criticism.

## PATIENT PERCEPTION OF THERAPIST BEHAVIOR

Two rating scales were used to measure the patient's attitudes toward the therapist and the patient's perception of the therapist's behavior. The first of these, the Relationship Questionnaire, was designed by Truax and Carkhuff to measure the patient's perception of therapist variables similar to those rated from tape recordings of the therapy sessions. The scale consists of four subscales and an overall measure. As can be seen in Figure 27, there were no statistically significant differences between patients' perception of behavior therapists and psychotherapists on accurate empathy, nonpossessive warmth, or concreteness. Behavior therapists were rated higher than psychotherapists on the genuineness (therapist self-congruence), and the overall scales, which was in keeping with the independent ratings made from tape recordings.

Second, Lorr's scale was used.[5] This is an inventory of 65 items designed to identify the main ways that clients perceive

Figure 27

Patients' Ratings of Therapists on the Relationship Questionnaire

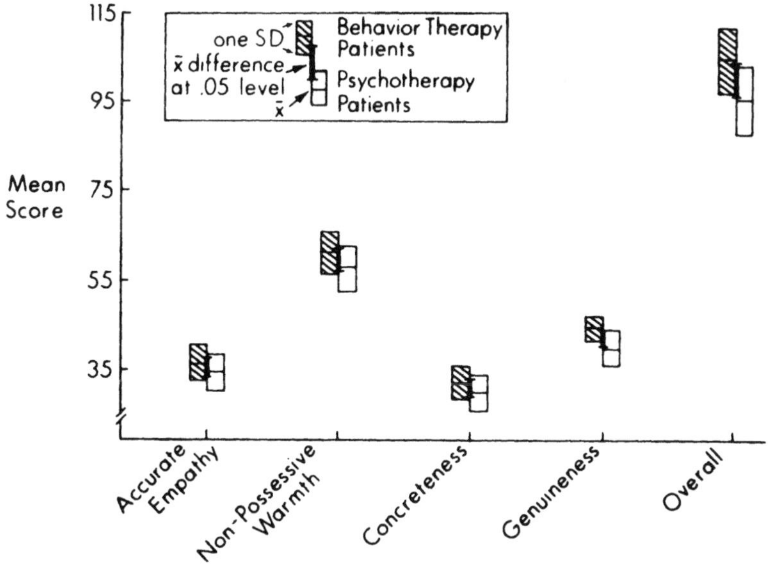

Figure 28

Patient Rating of Therapist Behavior (Lorr Scale)

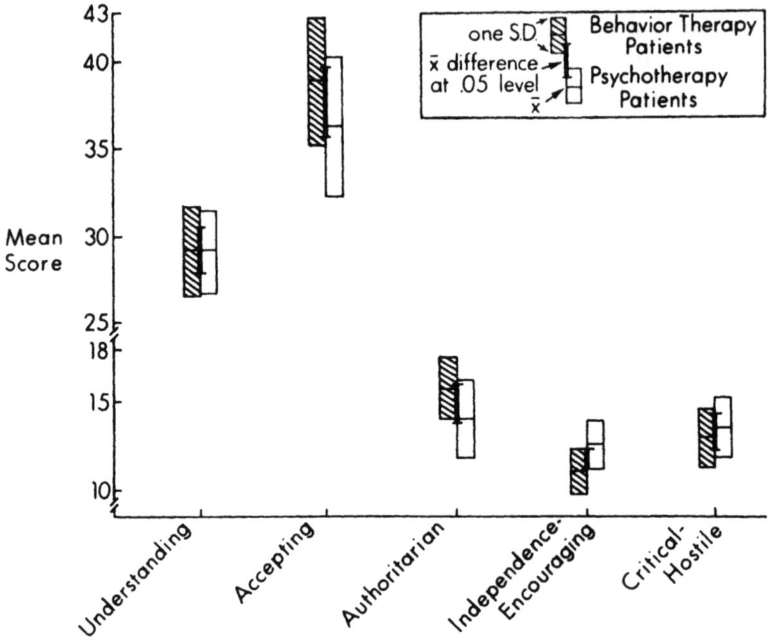


their therapists; these items represent five factors derived from a factor analysis of a larger pool of items. The factors are: understanding, accepting, authoritarian, independence-encouraging, and critical-hostile. All patients completed this scale at the end of four months' therapy. The results are shown in Figure 28.

The first factor, Understanding, is defined by behavior that indicates that the therapist understands what the patient is communicating and what he is feeling. Understanding would seem similar to Truax's "accurate empathy". There was no difference between the two groups of therapists on this factor.

The second factor, labeled Accepting by Lorr, consists of items related to interest and equalitarianism on the part of the therapist. Again there was no difference between the groups of therapists with respect to this variable.

Items in the third, "Authoritarian" scale relate to the patient's perception of the therapist as offering advice, direction, and assistance in reaching decisions. The expectation that behavior therapists would be rated higher than psychotherapists on this dimension was supported only at a marginal level of statistical significance. Objective ratings of therapy transcripts indicated that behavior therapists controlled the content of the conversation to a greater extent and gave more specific advice than did psychotherapists. However, such differences were apparently not as consistently perceived by patients.

The fourth factor, Independence-Encouraging, reflects the patient's view of how much his therapist encourages him to be independent. Psychotherapists were rated higher than behavior therapists on this scale.

In the final factor, labeled Critical-Hostile by Lorr, the patient perceives his therapist as critical, cold, impatient, and even competitive and disapproving. Again there were no significant differences between ratings of the two groups of therapists.

It was somewhat surprising in view of the marked differences between the two groups of therapists (in the analysis of tape recordings and transcripts of therapeutic interviews) that there were so few group differences in patients' perception of therapist behavior. One possibility, as suggested by Truax, is that patient questionnaires are less sensitive measures than the scales used in analyses of tape recordings. Another possibility is that patients simply do not notice the significant differences which objective raters perceived on these variables.

## DIFFERENCES AMONG INDIVIDUAL THERAPISTS

We have presented overall differences between behavior therapists and psychotherapists. In doing so, we gave only passing reference to the question of whether average differences might have resulted from unusually high or low scores by one or two therapists in each group. The question is partially answered by the significant differences found between groups, since significance is determined by group consistency as well as the size of the mean difference. Fiedler found, however, that experienced therapists of different persuasions resembled each other more than they resembled inexperienced therapists of their own schools; this effect could have been present here as well. [6]

In general, we found a remarkable degree of similarity among the three therapists within each group. The mean scores of each individual therapist in the higher-ranking group were clearly higher than the mean scores of each therapist in the other group when significant group differences were found. One therapist might be rated somewhat higher or lower than others, but the rank order remained consistent. The exception was average speech time.

A single therapist with deviant ratings contributed most to significant intergroup differences on the Truax ratings. It will be recalled that behavior therapists were rated higher than psychotherapists on depth of interpersonal contact, accurate empathy, and therapist self-congruence but not on unconditional positive regard. Figure 29 shows the means and standard deviations of the six therapists on these measures. One psychotherapist was consistently rated lower than his

Figure 29

Truax Ratings of Individual Therapists

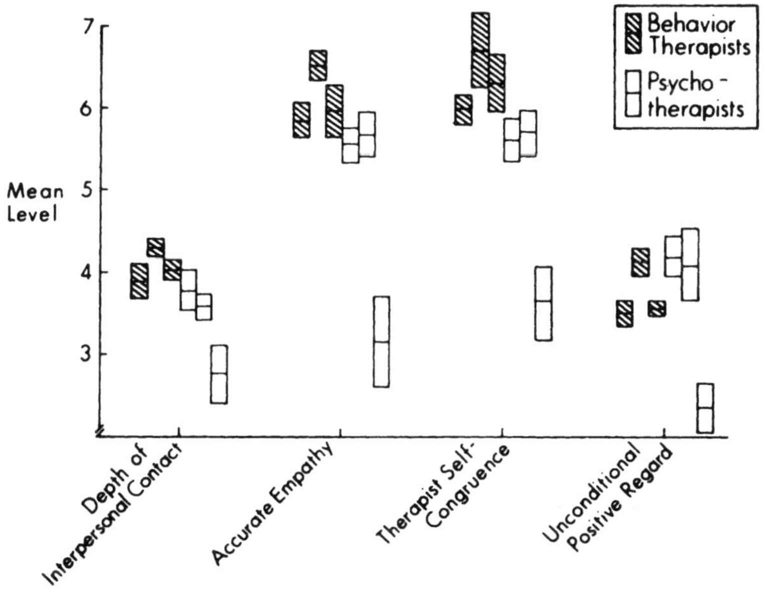


fellows on all four variables, and contributed heavily to the significant differences. However, there is some justification for the conclusion that behavior therapists as a group showed higher levels of these factors, since all behavior therapists were rated higher (albeit only slightly) than any of the psychotherapists. The ranking was not consistent for unconditional positive regard, where there was no significant difference between groups.

Differences between junior and senior therapists were not marked. The main difference was that senior therapists of both schools felt more of their patients were suitable for their treatment than did junior therapists.

## CLINICAL TECHNIQUES

As the patients' problems widely varied, so did the specific methods used to treat them. Each therapist used different strategies with different patients. The following description is compiled from each therapist's description to the assessor of how he treated each patient, verified by transcripts of recorded therapy sessions.

### *Psychotherapy*

The psychotherapists emphasized the importance of the therapy relationship, viewing it as the most important single factor in therapeutic success. In their descriptions of each patient's therapy, the therapists expressed this both directly ("developed a good relationship", "established emotional contact") and indirectly ("provided patient with a good father figure", "tried to show I was a warm, empathic person with whom she could talk").

The next most important factor, related to the first, was described by the words supportive, encouraging, reassuring. Having established such a relationship, the therapist encouraged the patient to explore and express feelings, guided the patient's introspection, and often contributed insights into his personality and the meaning of his feelings. Here the therapist's analytic orientation became obvious: abreaction, "softening of superego", uncovering repressions, free associations, and analysis of dreams and fantasies were mentioned as important and were clearly present in therapy transcripts. However, these did not seem really central to the progress of therapy. It seemed that a positive relationship was most important; second were discussion and (not exclusively analytical) insight and interpretation. Specific psychoanalytic techniques, although still important, were third.

The word advice was not used once in the psychotherapists'

description of their techniques, although there were in the transcripts rare instances of coaching on how to handle specific problems. These three therapists were very similar in their descriptions of treatment methods. The senior psychotherapist used psychoanalytic terms in his descriptions somewhat more often than did his junior colleagues, but this difference was not reflected in the therapy transcripts.

*Behavior Therapy*

There was more variation among the three behavior therapists' methods but, appropriately, all of them placed major emphasis on behavior modification. Classical behavior therapy techniques—relaxation training, systematic desensitization, aversive conditioning, assertive training—were used to an important extent by all three, and almost exclusively by the senior therapist. Role playing (behavioral rehearsal) was important to all of them. The second behavior therapist emphasized "cognitive restructuring" more than the others; his style was more didactic and discussion and insight were rather more important to him. Even here, and indeed wherever the behavior therapists turned from conditioning methods to methods seemingly more oriented toward insight, the accent remained on changing *behavior*. Discussions of feelings and their causes occurred much less often than discussions of maladaptive behaviors and how they could best be changed. Advice was often given. Reassurance and support were occasionally mentioned, but nearly always in conjunction with active behavioral measures. Similarly, behavior therapists occasionally specified trying to form a good relationship, but in only one or two cases was this at all central to the therapy. Generally, if considered at all, it was seen as a prerequisite to be achieved before beginning the real work of therapy.

## CONCLUSIONS

The data in this chapter clearly support the proposition that two quite separate and distinct treatments were given by therapists in this study. Differences between treatments were not only subjectively obvious but quantifiable on several dimensions as well. Principal differences were these:

Behavior therapists were more directive than psychotherapists. They more frequently gave explicit advice and instructions, provided information, and presented their own value judgments. They also exerted greater control over the content of the interaction by introducing new topics and seeking information. Psychotherapists played a more reflective role, allowing patients to select the topic of conversation and encouraging them to explore and express their thoughts and feelings. At times they showed the patient the mechanism of his problem and freed him to find his own solution. Only rarely did they let their personal opinions be perceived, much less put in the form of advice.

The more active role of behavior therapists was reflected in their speech patterns; they dominated the conversation to a much greater extent than did psychotherapists. On the average more of the therapeutic hour was taken up with therapists' speech rather than that of patients. By contrast, psychotherapists were more passive in the interview, allowing their patients roughly three times as much total speech time as they took themselves.

Psychotherapists placed much more emphasis on the therapeutic relationship. To our psychotherapists it does not much overstate the case to say that for many patients the personal relationship *was* the therapy. In nearly all cases it was the single most important factor, essential if psychotherapy was to succeed. Behavior therapists felt that in most cases a positive relationship was all that was necessary for therapy to proceed. A strong personal relationship was a welcome but not essential by-product of the therapists' understanding, nonjudgmental attitude, and little conscious effort was spent seeking it.

Curiously, the behavior therapists showed higher levels on the Truax scales of depth of interpersonal contact, therapist self-congruence, and accurate empathy in the fifth interview recordings. Both groups showed similar levels of unconditional positive regard or warmth toward patients. At first glance, this would suggest that behavior therapists were providing a closer and more effective relationship with the patient. However, these differences, particularly in depth of interpersonal contact and therapist self-congruence, may be more related to the style of the relationship than to its depth or effectiveness. Behavior therapists tended to respond to direct questions about themselves and the treatment, and allowed their personal feelings to be perceived by their patients. Psychotherapists tended to reflect direct questions and to reveal less of themselves while maintaining a more "professional" role during therapy. Behavior therapists might thus appear more "intimate" and "natural" with patients than did psychotherapists, but both showed an equal degree of unconditional warmth in the relationship. Of course, a behavior therapist might see his *conditional* positive regard as far more useful to appropriately reinforce the patient.

Psychotherapists were more directly concerned with feelings and their causes than with specific behaviors and means of changing them, while the opposite was true for behavior therapists. Obviously this only considers therapeutic strategies. As far as long-range goals are concerned, it was of course important to both that their patients should both feel well and act in adaptive ways.

Both theories and specific techniques differed widely. Psychotherapists thought in terms of psychoanalytic theory, behavior therapists in terms of learning theory. Psychotherapists used psychoanalytic techniques like free association and dream and fantasy analysis, behavior therapists used techniques like systematic desensitization and aversive conditioning.

In general, our analysis of the two therapies produced few surprises. Both groups behaved in therapy much as they said they did. While there was some diversity within each group, there were clear and consistent differences between the groups in therapeutic style, techniques, and pattern of interaction with the patient.

It is interesting that, despite these differences, treatment outcomes are essentially similar. This suggests that the temple of truth may be approached by different pathways, and that the treatments use two quite different approaches to reach the same end. Another possibility is that the treatments may be essentially similar along whatever dimensions actually contribute to change, but may differ on our measures, which may prove to tap only superficial aspects of therapy. Certainly it is difficult to counter the argument that some common factor just beyond empirical grasp is responsible for therapeutic change, particularly when the treatments share many features characteristic of individual therapy. This question is faced in the next chapter.

# 7 Patient Characteristics, Process Measures, and Outcome

For years psychotherapists have tried to isolate the characteristics of patients who are most likely to respond to treatment. Traditional psychotherapists have developed certain guidelines for selection of patients based on clinical experience. Research studies have found an enormous number of factors related to staying in treatment and to eventual therapeutic change.[1, 2, 3] Most of these studies are unreplicated and their variables are of dubious validity.

In this chapter we will discuss, first, what patient characteristics are related to improvement and second, what aspects of treatment appear responsible for success. First we will be concerned with whether patients with certain characteristics respond more favorably to one form of treatment than another.

With the data available from the present study we asked a number of specific questions. First, is one treatment more effective with certain patients than with others? For example, is behavior therapy more effective for patients with high levels of anxiety than for those with low levels? Is psychotherapy more effective with younger than with older patients? A second and related question is, which patients are most amenable to what form of treatment? Are anxious patients more effectively treated by behavior therapy than by psychotherapy? Is psychotherapy more effective than behavior therapy for patients with psychosomatic problems? Third, which untreated patients show improvement and which do not? Are there certain types of problems which improve spontaneously and others which do not? Or is the improvement shown by wait-list patients independent of the particular pathology involved?

A second general aim was to understand each therapy more fully by attempting to isolate critical aspects of each treatment. Many process and relationship factors have been shown to relate to success of treatment. Are the same factors related to success in behavior therapy as in analytically oriented psychotherapy? Put another way, is there some therapeutic process common to both treatments, regardless of therapist's expressed theoretical differences, or do both treatments result in patient improvement through entirely different procedures?

## OUTCOME MEASURES

Throughout this chapter we used a single index of improvement, a regression transformation of change scores of the target symptoms. This is described in detail in Appendix 6. The purpose of this transformation is to remove the restricting effect of original severity from the ratings of change in severity. To obtain a precise estimate of the contribution of each patient and therapist characteristic to therapeutic outcome, some form of multivariate analysis such as discriminant function analysis would be the most appropriate statistical technique. However, in the present study, such techniques were not used. We had initially decided to use as many measures of patient and process variables as seemed feasible—both to see how standard measures from the literature compared with our study and to add our own measures when it seemed appropriate. This led to a situation where there were more possible variables than number of observations or patients. Also, to use measures for their psychological importance rather than their statistical congruence would have meant combining data from interval, ordinal, and nominal scales. For these reasons we decided on an alternative technique.

In order to show graphically the relationship between each of the patient characteristics and therapeutic outcome, each group was divided into two on the basis of the median scores of each patient measure. Means and standard deviations of the target symptom improvement scores (T scores derived from the regression equation) were then calculated separately for the group that scored above the median and for the group that scored below the median on each patient measure at initial assessment. Thus, Figure 30 shows the means and standard deviations of improvement scores of patients in psychotherapy for those who initially scored high or low on each MMPI scale. The height of the bars plots the standard deviation, while the horizontal line in the middle of the bar represents the mean value for that subgroup. Thus, for the first scale the dotted bar represents the 15 patients who scored lowest on the hypochondriasis scale, with a mean outcome score of 54 and a standard deviation of 10 (plotted from 49 to 59 equidistant on either side of the mean). The heavy line between the two vertical bars represents the difference between the two means which would be required for statistical significance at the .05 level for a two-tailed test. Thus, if the heavy line in the center does not overlap the horizontal lines representing the means, a significant difference between the two groups is indicated. If the heavy line does overlap the means, there is no statistically significant difference between the high and low groups.

Statistical significance in this sense must be interpreted cautiously. Because of the large number of significance tests which will be performed in this way, a certain number would be expected to reach significance through the operation of chance factors alone. However, these differences in the means which would be required to reach statistical significance are plotted in order to make the reliability of the differences between groups readily apparent to visual inspection. Since this part of the study is basically a "hypothesis suggesting" rather than a "hypothesis testing" procedure, the practice was felt to be justified.

## PATIENT CHARACTERISTICS: MMPI

Those patients who initially scored low on the Minnesota Multiphasic Personality Inventory scales tended to show greater target symptom improvement with psychotherapy than those who scored high (Figure 30). Conversely, those patients who scored high on the hysteria and psychopathic deviate scales, which often reflect antisocial, acting-out behavior, did significantly less well than those who scored low. Both these findings support clinical impressions: first that insight psychotherapy is most effective with patients who are less severely disturbed and second that patients who act out their problems do less well than those who are bothered by the internal suffering of ego-dystonic symptoms.

In contrast, behavior therapy was equally successful whether the patient had a high or low degree of pathology (Figure 31). Moreover, behavior therapy patients with initially high levels of hysteria and mania improved *more* than those who were low. This suggests that those patients who are characterized by antisocial acting-out tendencies are less amenable to psychotherapy but more amenable to behavior therapy.

There were no consistent or significant differences in the wait-list group (Figure 32). There was a tendency for the patients who scored lower on the MMPI scales to show greater

Figure 30

MMPI and Treatment Outcome for Psychotherapy Patients

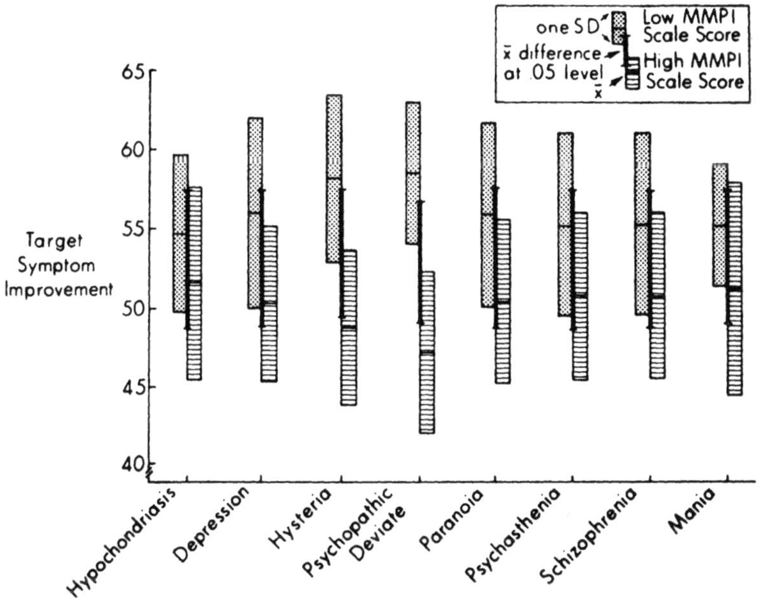


improvement than those who scored initially higher. The one exception was those patients who were initially more depressed; they showed slightly greater improvement than those who were initially less so.

Figure 33 compares the success of the three treatments with patients with high pathology on each of the MMPI scales. With the exception of the high-depression patients, both treated groups clearly showed greater improvement than did wait-list patients. Thus short-term "talking" therapies were less effective for depressed patients (as judged by the MMPI) than for others.

As was expected from the within-treatment comparisons,

Figure 31

MMPI and Treatment Outcome for Behavior Therapy Patients

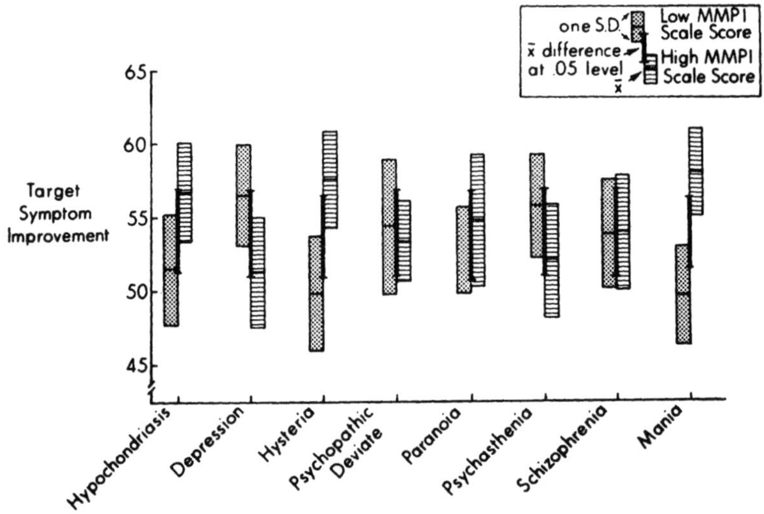


differences between behavior therapy and psychotherapy were most evident on the hysteria, psychopathic deviate, and mania scales. Behavior therapy tended to be the more effective treatment for these syndromes, although differences reached statistical significance only in the case of hysteria.

## DEGREE OF INITIAL DISTURBANCE

There was a strong, though nonsignificant, tendency for psychotherapy patients who had more initial pathology on work and social scales not to improve as much as those who had less. These trends were not as evident for behavior therapy patients. Initial target symptom severity was not significantly related to outcome for either group (Figure 34).

There was a clear relationship between treatment outcome

Figure 32

MMPI and Treatment Outcome for Wait List Patients

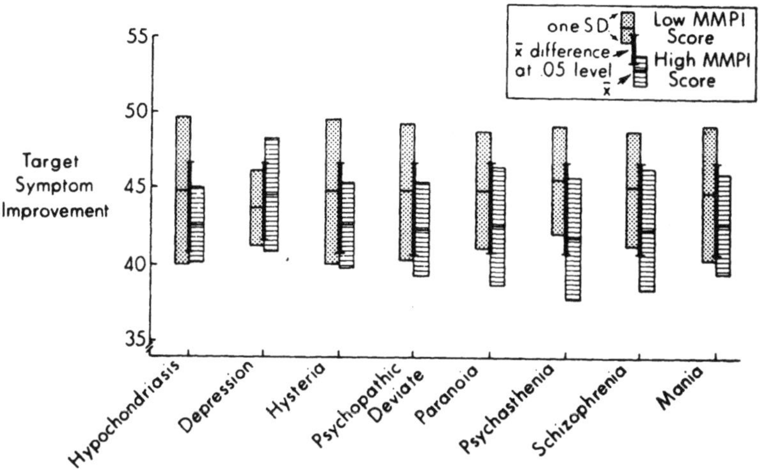


and degree of initial disturbance when the disturbance was measured by the patient's own report (MMPI). There was less relationship with outcome when independent ratings of work and social pathology and target symptom severity were used. Truax and Carkhuff have emphasized the distinction between dynamic or "felt" aspects and symptomatic or "overt" aspects of patient pathology.[4] They suggested that therapeutic gain should be greatest with the combination of high "felt" and low "overt" disturbance; least with low "felt" and high "overt" disturbance. We measured "felt" disturbance by the MMPI mean scale elevation. This is the average of all clinical scales except masculinity-femininity and social introversion. The questionnaire allows patients to register a wide range of complaints reflecting their subjective discomfort. We used

Figure 33

Treatment Outcome for Patients with High Initial MMPI Scores

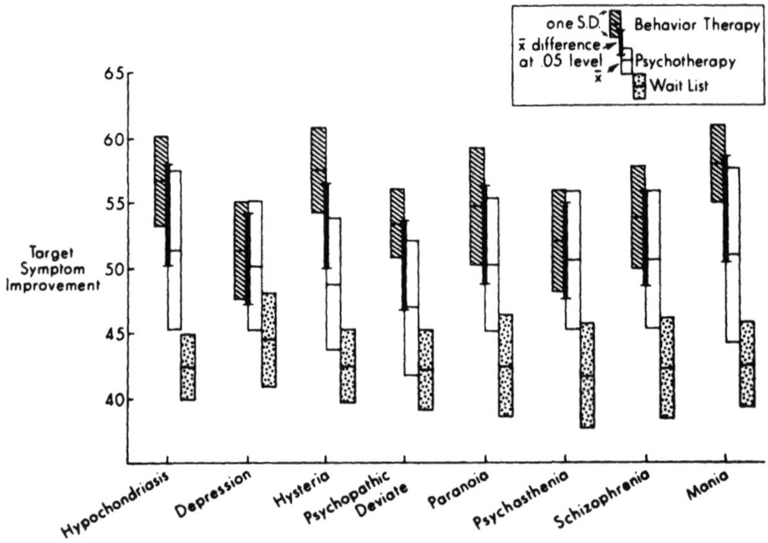


severity of target symptoms to measure overt disturbance. Again these were voiced complaints (like all symptoms) but quantified by the independent assessors.

Four subgroups of patients were formed for each treatment group by splitting the groups at the median on each measure, taking as "high" those above and as "low" those below the median. Since the relationship between each of these variables and outcome differed for the behavior therapy and psychotherapy patients, separate analyses were performed for each treatment group. Mean improvement scores for patients with severe symptoms-high MMPI, severe symptoms-low MMPI, moderate symptoms-high MMPI and moderate symptoms-low MMPI are in Figure 35.

Psychotherapy patients with high initial disturbance showed

Figure 34

Treatment Outcome and Initial Level of Severity

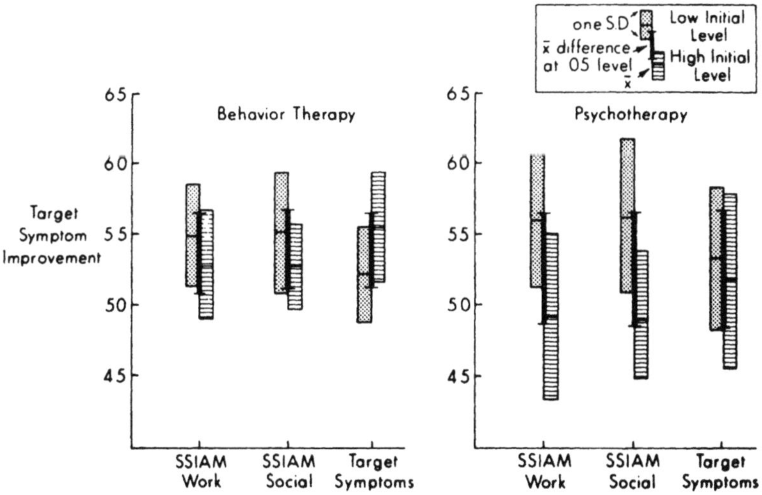


less improvement than those with low disturbance ($F = 5.19$, $p < .05$). However, the significant symptom x MMPI interaction effect ($F = 5.55$, $p < .05$) indicates that this effect was most marked for patients with high initial pathology on both MMPI and target symptoms. Such patients showed significantly less improvement than any of the other psychotherapy groups when mean differences were tested by Duncan's Multiple Range Test. Thus patients who complained the most and had the most disturbance got least help from psychotherapy. There were no significant differences among behavior therapy subgroups. In both treatment groups, patients who were low in felt disturbance and high in overt disturbance tended to improve most. Thus our findings did not support Truax's prediction. Other studies that have examined this relationship have obtained inconsistent and contradictory results.[5]

Figure 35

Treatment Outcome and Severity of Initial Disturbance

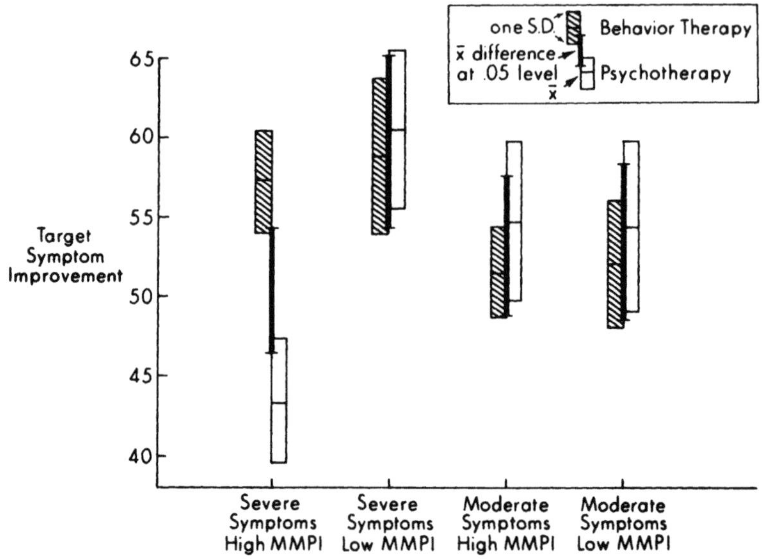


Clearly, however, the relationship is heavily influenced by the criteria used for "overt" pathology, the outcome measures, and their relationship to felt disturbance and how it is defined.

## PERSONALITY CHARACTERISTICS

Symptomatic improvement of psychotherapy patients scoring high and low on the extraversion and neuroticism scales of the Eysenck Personality Inventory, the self-acceptance, self-control, sociability, and socialization scales of the California Psychological Inventory and the social introversion and Taylor Manifest Anxiety Scale from the MMPI are shown in Figure 36. There were no consistent or reliable differences among those patients scoring high or low. However, there was a tendency toward more improvement in patients who were better adjus-

Figure 36

Personality Measures and Treatment Outcome: Psychotherapy Patients

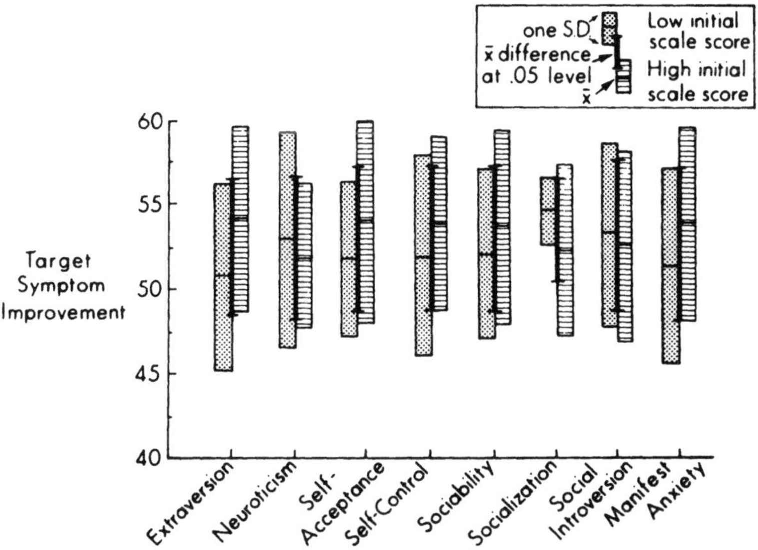


ted in the sense of showing higher self-acceptance and self-control, greater sociability, and less neuroticism. These findings did not provide positive support for the hypothesis that less severely disturbed patients improved more with insight psychotherapy, but they were consistent with this notion.

There were no marked or consistent differences in outcome related to patient personality characteristics for the behavior therapy (Figure 37) or wait-list patients (Figure 38). DiLoreto [6] and others have suggested that introverted patients should show greater improvement than extraverted patients with systematic desensitization, one of behavior therapy's major techniques. Our data do not directly test this hypothesis, since systematic desensitization was not used with every patient.

Figure 37

Personality Measures and Treatment Outcome: Behavior Therapy Patients

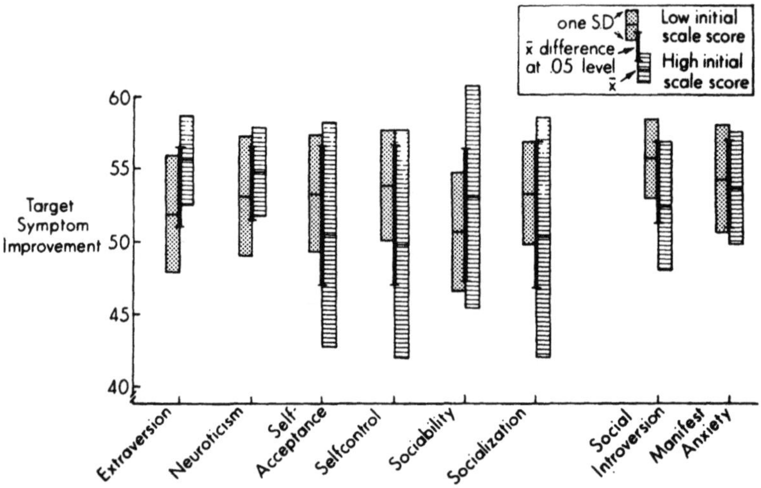


Figure 38

Personality Measures and Treatment Outcome: Wait List Patients

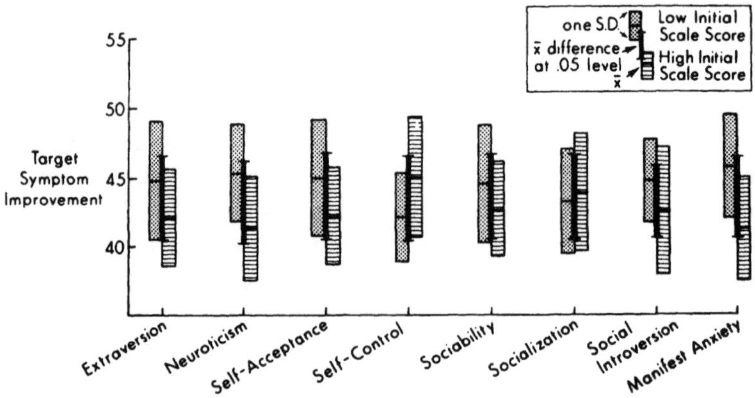

Still, the data here are not consistent with this notion. There was, in fact, a tendency for introverted patients to improve less than extraverted patients in behavior therapy, when extraversion was assessed either by the MMPI or by the Eysenck Personality Inventory.

The personality characteristics did not predict which patients respond better to which kind of treatment. As shown in Figure 39, patients who were introverted, extraverted, anxious, neurotic, self-accepting, self-controlled, sociable, and highly socialized responded equally well to behavior therapy or analytically oriented psychotherapy, and less well to a minimal-contact treatment.

Figure 39

Outcome for Patients with High Scores on Selected Personality Characteristics

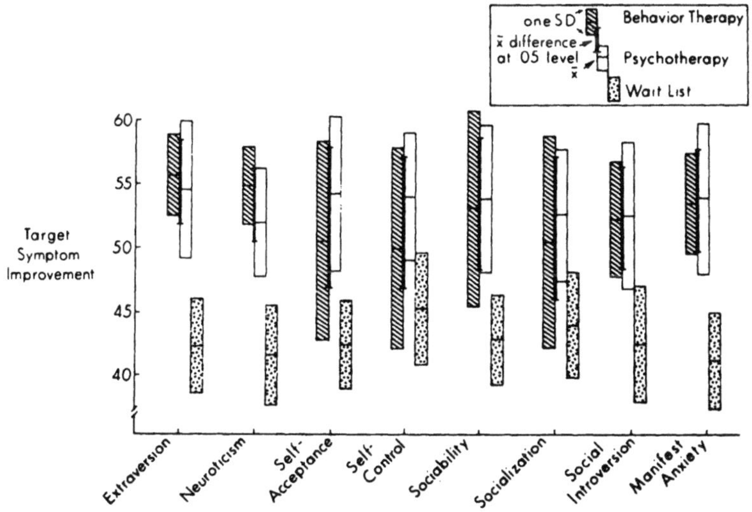

## TARGET SYMPTOMS

Average improvement scores for each kind of symptom represent the difference between that symptom's initial severity and its four-month severity rating. These are presented in Figure 40, for each context of symptom in Figure 41, and for each mode of action of symptom in Figure 42. Because there were so few symptoms in several categories, no attempt was made to perform statistical tests on these data. In Figure 40, which presents outcome according to the kind of symptom, there is little overlap among the treated and untreated groups. Both the behavior therapy and psychotherapy patients clearly showed greater improvement than wait-list patients, with little difference between the two treated groups. The only overlap be-

Figure 40

Kinds of Symptoms and Treatment Outcome

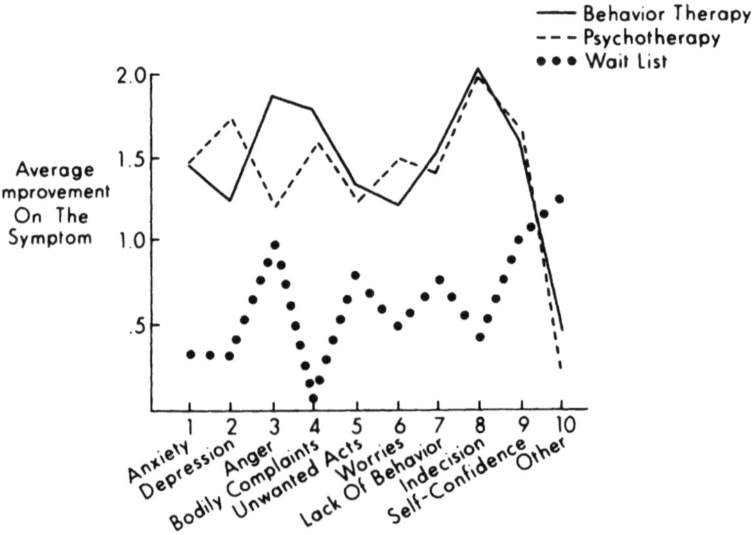

Figure 41

Contexts of Symptoms and Treatment Outcome

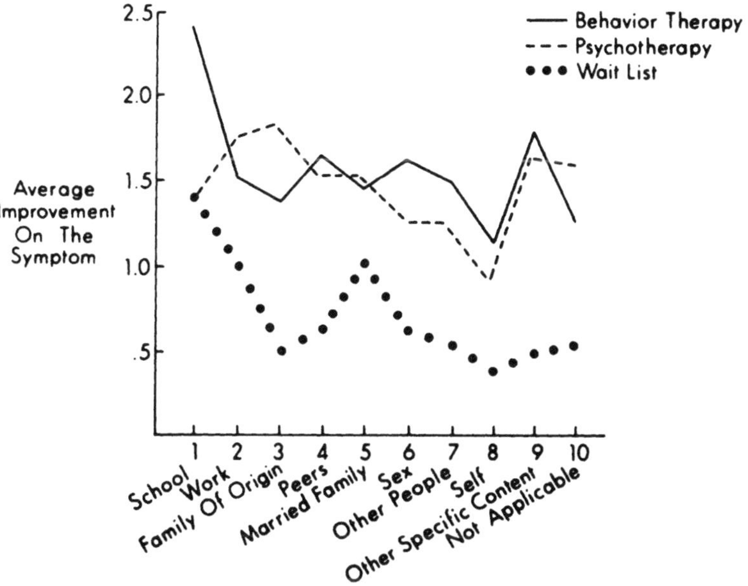


tween the wait-list and the treated groups is in the "other," or miscellaneous, category. In all other areas, both treated groups improved more than the wait list, with no significant difference between the two treated groups. Also for the context and mode of action of symptoms, both treated groups appeared similar but markedly different from the wait-list group (Figures 41 and 42). These three graphs, Figures 40, 41, and 42, are remarkably similar in the sense that neither behavior therapy nor psychotherapy was more effective with one specific symptom than another, and both were consistently more effective than the minimal-contact treatment represented by the wait list.

Figure 42

Modes of Action of Symptoms and Treatment Outcome

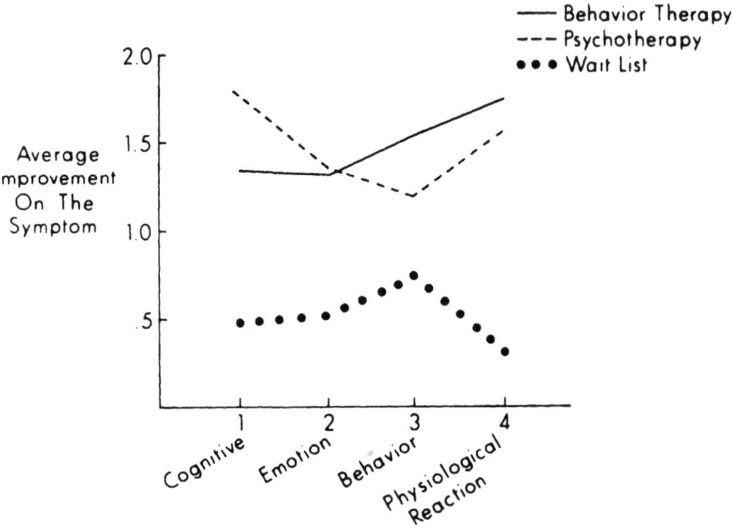


## DEMOGRAPHIC CHARACTERISTICS AND OUTCOME

The relationship between demographic characteristics and therapeutic outcome was examined to see if it differed among the three treatments. Table 23 shows means and standard deviations of outcome scores for groups formed from the following characteristics: age (high or low, based on median split), sex, married (yes or no), number of siblings (high or low, based on a median split of number of siblings), education (high or low, based on a median split of years of education), income (high or low, based on median split), birth order (first-born or later-born), and intelligence (high or low, based on a median split of Mill Hill scores).

There were no significant differences in outcome related to sex, age, marital status, number of siblings, education, birth

TABLE 23. Demographic Characteristics and Outcome

| | Behavior Therapy | | Psychotherapy | | Wait List | |
|---|---|---|---|---|---|---|
| Age | High | Low | High | Low | High | Low |
| Mean outcome | 52.07 | 55.00 | 51.43 | 53.33 | 43.19 | 43.62 |
| S.D. | 7.62 | 6.35 | 10.45 | 11.27 | 9.10 | 6.59 |
| Sex | Male | Female | Male | Female | Male | Female |
| Mean outcome | 54.58 | 53.44 | 49.67 | 54.50 | 42.25 | 44.33 |
| S.D. | 8.99 | 5.76 | 11.23 | 9.97 | 8.38 | 7.56 |
| Married | Yes | No | Yes | No | Yes | No |
| Mean outcome | 51.50 | 54.77 | 55.71 | 51.61 | 44.44 | 43.10 |
| S.D. | 7.39 | 6.97 | 8.63 | 11.16 | 7.72 | 8.04 |
| Number of siblings | High | Low | High | Low | High | Low |
| Mean outcome | 53.33 | 54.28 | 49.21 | 55.50 | 43.78 | 43.08 |
| S.D. | 7.51 | 6.99 | 11.23 | 9.43 | 7.35 | 8.79 |
| Education | High | Low | High | Low | High | Low |
| Mean outcome | 55.17 | 53.06 | 54.07 | 50.63 | 44.63 | 42.21 |
| S.D. | 6.46 | 7.51 | 12.59 | 8.91 | 7.89 | 7.86 |
| Income | High | Low | High | Low | High | Low |
| Mean outcome | 53.47 | 55.36 | 57.43 | 47.18 | 40.15 | 46.64 |
| S.D. | 6.97 | 7.78 | 8.06 | 11.29 | 8.57 | 6.18 |
| First-born | Yes | No | Yes | No | Yes | No |
| Mean outcome | 53.00 | 55.64 | 53.11 | 56.80 | 44.42 | 42.89 |
| S.D. | 7.14 | 7.29 | 9.17 | 10.30 | 10.63 | 5.43 |
| Intelligence | High | Low | High | Low | High | Low |
| Mean outcome | 53.73 | 54.07 | 55.38 | 50.07 | 43.00 | 44.93 |
| S.D. | 7.20 | 7.73 | 10.39 | 7.52 | 7.37 | 9.04 |

order, or intelligence for any of the treatments. Patients with high income showed significantly greater improvement in psychotherapy than patients with low income. But wait-list patients with low income showed significantly greater improvement than wait-list patients with high income. In psychotherapy, relatively greater success was associated with being younger, female, married, late born, from a smaller family, with more education, income, and intelligence. Although these results were not statistically significant, they were much more marked and consistent for psychotherapy than for behavior therapy. They were in keeping with clinical notions of suitable psychotherapeutic patients. Overall, our sample of patients was a fairly homogeneous group, being primarily young, single, with high educational status, and considered good candidates for psychotherapy. Greater differences among these demographic characteristics might have been shown with a sample more representative of the total population.

With this discussion we leave measures of patient characteristics and turn to process measures.

## PROCESS MEASURES: TRUAX RATINGS

There was no relationship between Truax variables and outcome in either active therapy (Figures 43 and 44). This is somewhat surprising in view of the many studies cited by Truax which suggest that the levels of interpersonal contact, accurate empathy, therapist self-congruence, and unconditional positive regard offered by the therapist are critical for success of treatment. However, with one exception,[7] most of these involve some form of Rogerian or nondirective therapy, in contrast to the psychoanalytically oriented and behavior therapy of our study. Relatively few deal with therapists comparable to ours. Garfield and Bergin[8] found no relationship between these variables and outcome for therapists "who were largely outside the client-centered orientation," and the one

Figure 43

Truax Variables and Treatment Outcome: Psychotherapy Patients

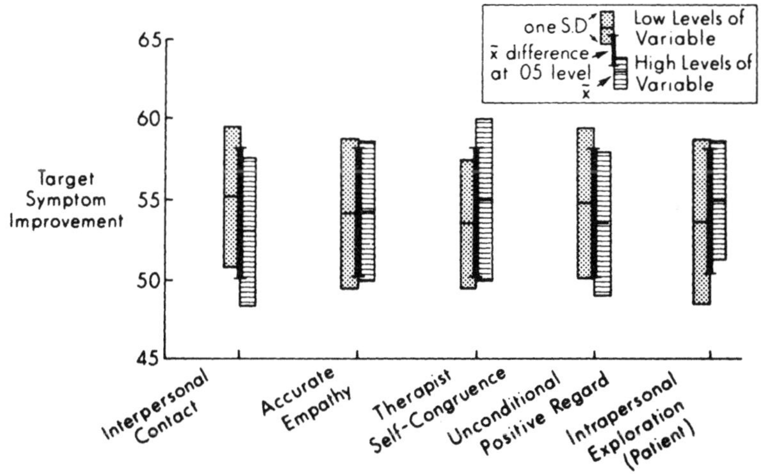


Figure 44

Truax Variables and Treatment Outcome:
Behavior Therapy Patients

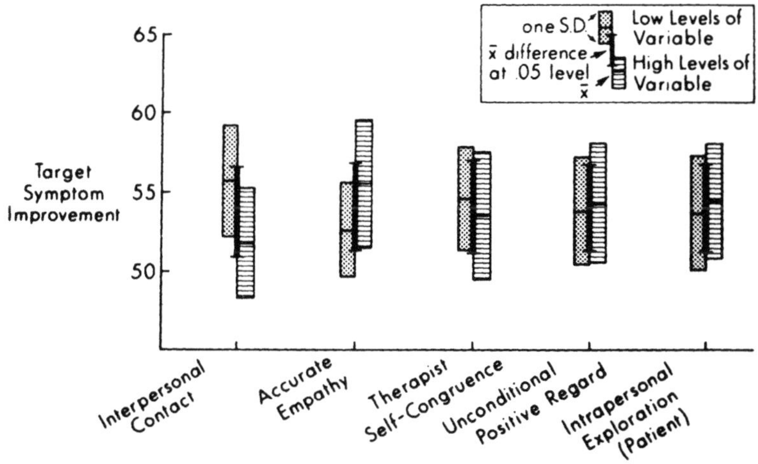

study by Truax *et al.*[9] with analytically oriented therapists was not conclusive.

It may be that these factors, or at least the specific scales used to measure them, are not relevant for other therapeutic orientations. Another possible explanation is that therapists in the Truax study were beginners who were by no means expert in their application of treatment. The level of the factors offered was lower than that provided by the experienced therapists of our study. Consequently, differences between high and low levels of these factors would not be as marked in our study and there would be less opportunity for differences in outcome to emerge. Similarly, few patients got worse. Presumably all our psychotherapists had adequate levels of interpersonal skills to avoid the deterioration effects claimed to be most common at the hands of psychonoxious psychotherapists.[10]

It is curious to note that "depth of intrapersonal exploration" of the patient was not related to outcome. Patients who discussed their problems on a "more meaningful" level showed no more improvement than did those who discussed their problems in a more superficial way. This scale has previously been used to measure "openness to therapeutic influence." But our results did not support the hypothesis that patient openness to influence is an important prognostic indicator.

With behavior therapy the only factor which approached statistical significance was that of interpersonal contact, and this was opposite to prediction. That is, patients whose therapists showed less interpersonal contact tended to show greater improvement than those whose therapists showed higher levels. It will be recalled that behavior therapists showed significantly higher levels of interpersonal contact, accurate empathy, and therapist self-congruence than did psychotherapists. Although these variables differentiated therapists in this study, they did not predict the outcome of treatment.

## PATIENT SPEECH CHARACTERISTICS

Patients who spoke more in therapy, that is, those who showed greater total speech time, did better in psychotherapy than those who spoke less (Fig. 45). Such patients did not speak more often but rather spoke in longer blocks when they did speak. There was also a tendency for successful patients to react more quickly to the therapist's comments, as the difference between high and low reaction times approached statistical significance. These results are consistent with a previous study of analytically oriented short-term psychotherapy.[21] They are also consistent with the image of a good psychotherapy patient as one who is talkative, who speaks in longer and more complete thought units, and who reacts more

Figure 45

Speech Characteristics and Treatment Outcome: Psychotherapy Patients

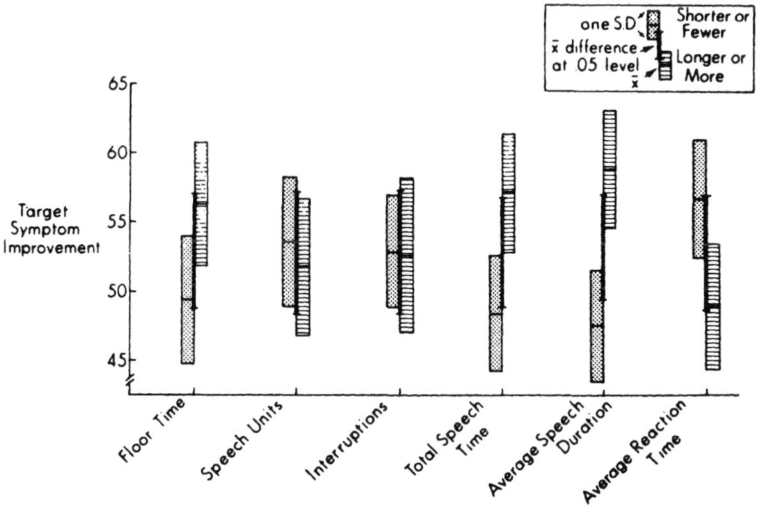

quickly to the therapist's comments, and consequently allows shorter silences.

With behavior therapy, differences between successful and less successful patients were not as marked, as is shown in Fig. 46. Patients who spoke in longer utterances showed statistically greater improvement in therapy than those who spoke in shorter blocks. As this relationship held for both active treatments it appears a general predictor of therapeutic outcome. However, neither the total speech time of the patients nor their average reaction time was related to success in behavior therapy.

## LENNARD AND BERNSTEIN INFORMATIONAL SPECIFICITY RATINGS

There were no significant relationships between outcome and high and low levels of the therapist's rating on the Lennard and Bernstein specific interaction categories (Figures 47 and 48, Appendix 5). This was true for both active treatments. In

Figure 46

Speech Characteristics and Treatment Outcome: Behavior Therapy Patients

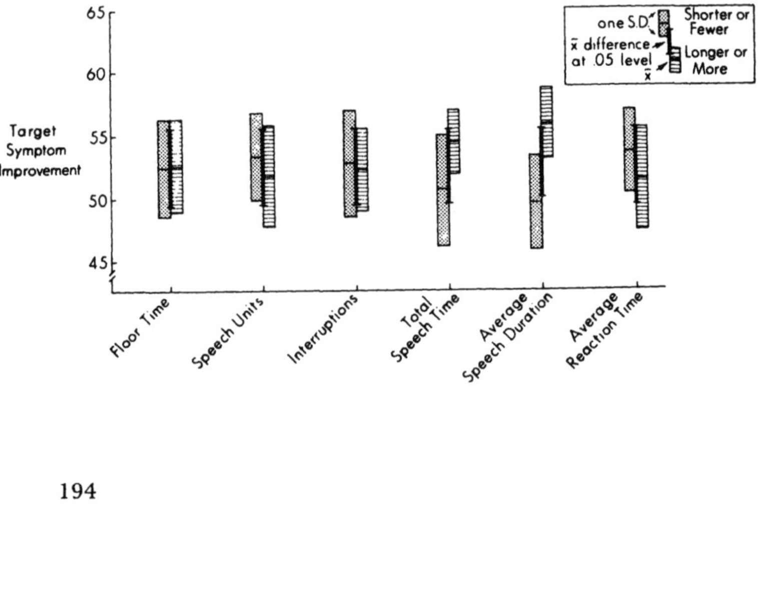

Figure 47

Therapist Informational Specificity
and Treatment Outcome: Psychotherapy Patients

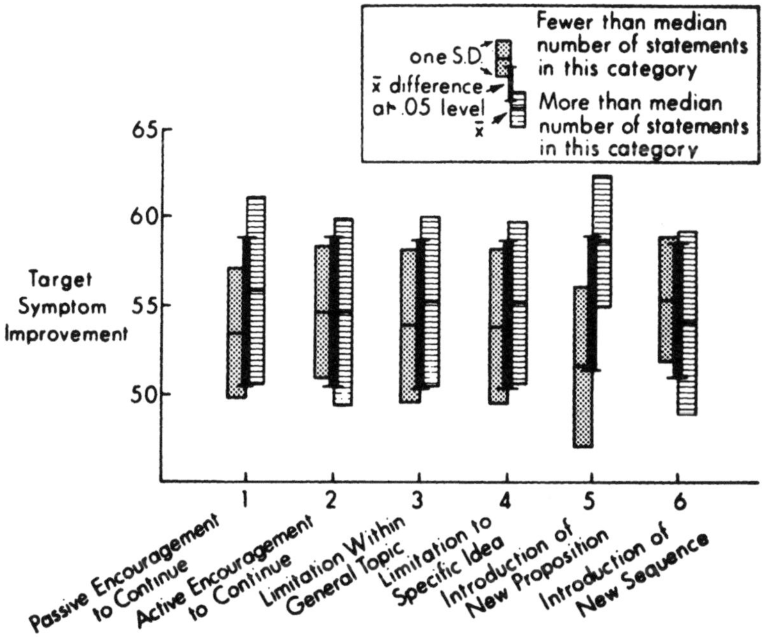


psychotherapy one category (number 5, referring to the frequency with which a therapist introduces a new proposition) approached statistical significance. There were too few requests for specific information by psychotherapists to make a meaningful comparison for this category. It will be recalled (Figure 21) that there were marked differences between behavior therapists and psychotherapists in the frequency with which they used these categories in therapy. Psychotherapists gave more statements indicating that their comments followed from the topics or content areas introduced by the patient,

Figure 48

Therapist Informational Specificity
and Treatment Outcome: Behavior Therapy Patients

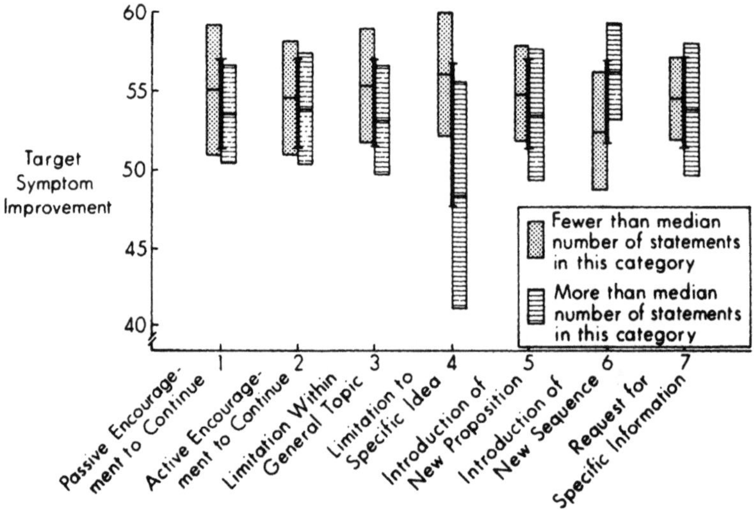


whereas behavior therapists more frequently introduced new content areas. However, these tendencies seemed to be simply a characteristic of each therapy and were not related to improvement.

## TEMPLE CONTENT CATEGORIES

The Temple Content Categories show that patients whose psychotherapists used fewer clarifying and interpretive statements showed greater improvement than those whose therapists used more (Figure 49, category 3). This rather paradoxical finding suggests that the more therapists attempted to clarify, interpret, and give psychological information directly related to the problem, the less successful the treatment. It is possible

Figure 49
Temple Content Categories and Treatment Outcome: Psychotherapy Patients

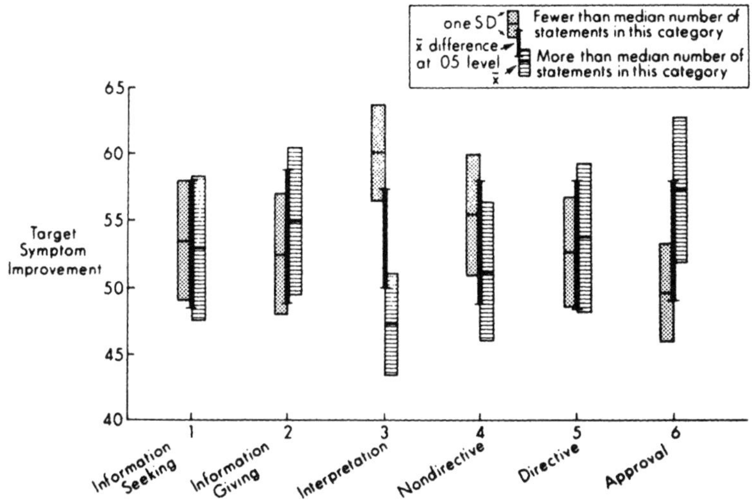


that psychotherapists, when faced with a patient who has little insight or inclination to look into psychological causes of his own behavior, may use more statements in this category in an attempt to stimulate the patient to think in these terms. In contrast the patients who were more psychologically minded, and usually considered more likely to improve, needed less interpretation. Conversely it is possible that interpretive statements may be valueless unless accepted by the patient. This we did not measure. Finally interpretive statements in general may do little good, despite the widespread belief in their value. Few specific studies have been made comparable to Malan's, in which he pointed to the value of the transference parent link to good outcome.[11] Only some of our psychotherapists' interpretive comments would fit his definition and our findings cannot be compared.

The only other category in which differences approached statistical significance was that of direct statements of approval. Patients whose therapists gave them more direct expressions of approval tended to show improved outcome. This probably arose from the tendency of therapists to reward or approve of patients' statements indicating some insight or modification of behavior and feelings in a therapeutic direction, i.e., conditional positive regard. The overall frequency of such statements was in fact fairly low and it is unlikely that such reward was used as a systematic motivation.

There were no significant differences for the behavior therapists (Figure 50). There was a tendency for therapists whose patients showed greater improvement to use more statements in category 7, that is, direct expressions of disapproval. However, such expressions were made infrequently and seem unlikely to have been a major factor in treatment. They were so rare in the psychotherapy group that no comparisons were made.

## THERAPIST ATTITUDE TOWARD THE PATIENT

Patients who were more liked by their psychotherapists showed greater improvement than those who were less liked (Figure 51). This suggests that the therapist's positive feeling toward the patient may be important for success in insight therapy, and tends to confirm the clinical belief that the relationship between patient and therapist is critical in analytically oriented psychotherapy. In addition, patients who more closely resembled the usual patients of their therapist (category 10) improved significantly more than patients who were less usual. There was also a tendency for patients who were con-

Figure 50

Temple Content Categories and Treatment Outcome: Behavior Therapy Patients

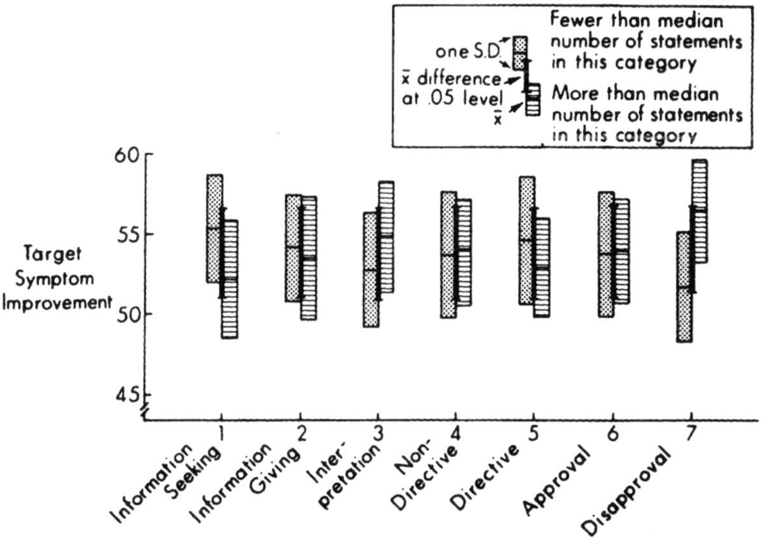


sidered more suitable for treatment to show greater improvement (category 2).

The therapist's liking for the patient did not appear related to success in behavior therapy (Figure 52, category 1). However, there was a tendency for patients with whom the therapist felt more comfortable (3) and whom he considered more interesting (9) to improve more. This suggests that the relationship between patient and therapist may also be important for success in behavior therapy but to a lesser extent than in psychotherapy.

One problem in the interpretation of these data is that ratings of patients were completed at the end of four months' therapy. The therapists' liking for the patient may have been

Figure 51

Psychotherapist Attitude Toward Patients and Treatment Outcome

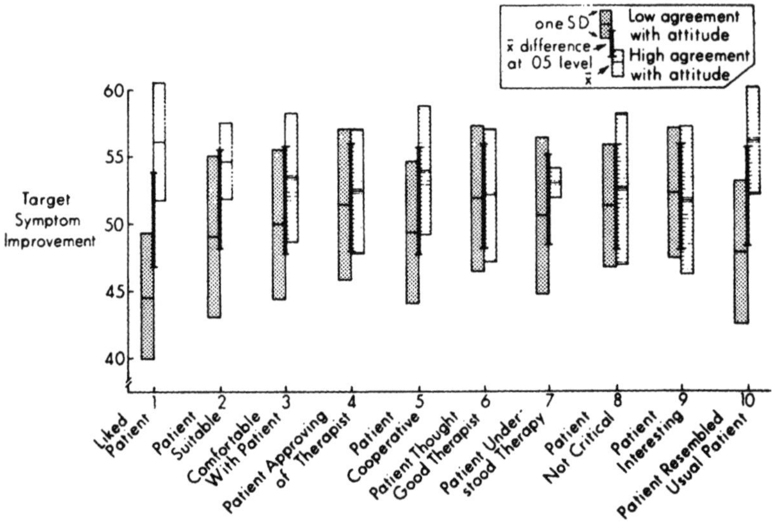


influenced by knowledge of how well the patient did in treatment. This bias is eliminated in some studies by having therapists rate patients at the beginning rather than at the end of treatment. However, such ratings, based on an immediate impression of the patient, perhaps do not mean as much as those made after considerable contact. Also, marked differences in outcome between patients who were more or less liked was evident only for the psychotherapy group. Such differences were not evident among behavior therapists.

## PATIENT PERCEPTION OF THE THERAPIST

Although no overall differences reached statistical significance, there was a strong tendency for patients who perceived a greater nonpossessive warmth and genuineness in their psychotherapists to improve more (Figure 53). Results were very similar for behavior therapy patients (Figure 54). No

Figure 52

Behavior Therapist Attitude Toward Patients and Treatment Outcome

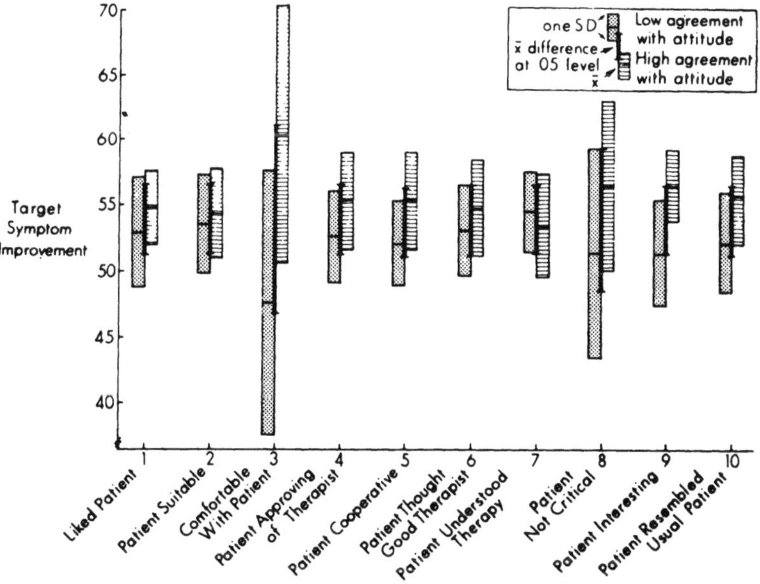


group differences reached statistical significance, but again there was a strong tendency for patients to improve more who perceived higher levels of nonpossessive warmth and accurate empathy.

These findings are compatible with the importance of the relationship in either type of therapy, but somewhat inconclusive.

Objective ratings of Truax factors made from taped interviews and from the patient questionnaires showed clear differences between behavior therapy and psychotherapy. Ratings made from the tapes by independent judges were not related to success of treatment. However, patients who showed greater improvement tended to see better therapeutic qualities in their therapists than those who improved less. Again, these

Figure 53

Relationship Questionnaire and Treatment Outcome: Psychotherapy Patients

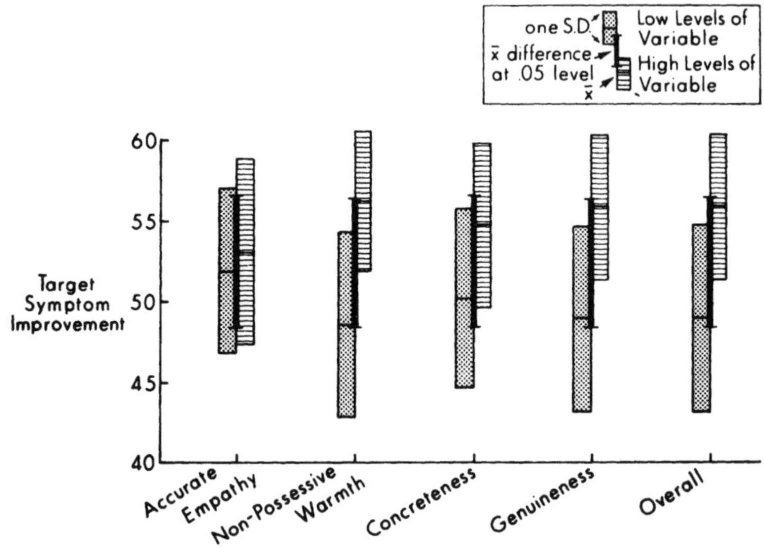


ratings were made after four months' treatment. The patients may have been biased toward seeing better therapeutic qualities in those who had helped them compared to those who had not.

On the Lorr the patient's perception of the therapist as understanding, authoritarian, independence-encouraging, or critical-hostile were not related to outcome (Figure 55). There was a nonsignificant tendency for both psychotherapy and behavior therapy patients who perceived their therapist as more accepting to show greater improvement (Figure 56).

## THE PATIENT'S PERCEPTION OF TREATMENT

Between one and two years after completing therapy, the patients were mailed a questionnaire which asked for their im-

Figure 54

Relationship Questionnaire and Treatment Outcome:
Behavior Therapy Patients

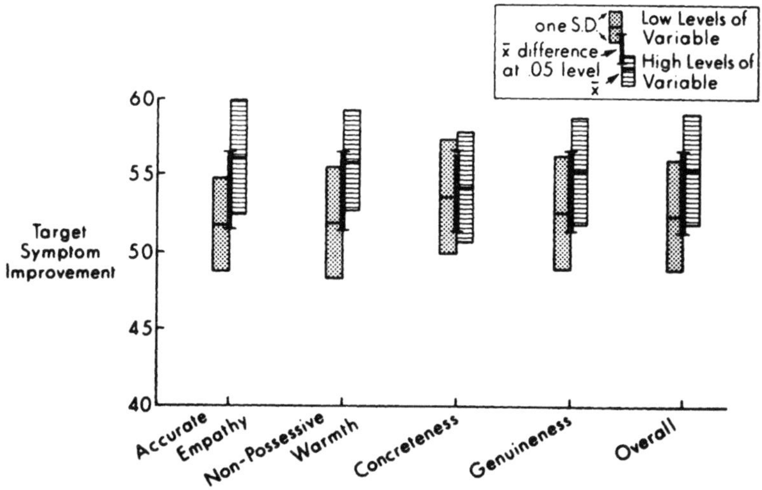


pressions of their treatment. Of the sixty treated patients, forty-eight (half behavior therapy and half insight therapy) patients returned their questionnaires. These patients were divided into three groups on the basis of their answers to the first question, which asked for a global rating of the helpfulness of treatment. Those who rated therapy as "extremely helpful" or "very helpful" were called successes; those who rated therapy as "slightly helpful" or "unhelpful" were failures, and "intermediate" patients found therapy "helpful." In the discussion that follows, intermediate patients' replies will mostly be omitted, in order the better to contrast the successes and failures of therapy. Of these there were 54% successes and 17% failures among the behavior therapy patients who replied, and 37% successes and 37% failures in the psychotherapy patients who did so. The difference was not statistically significant.

Figure 55

Patient Perception of Psychotherapist Behavior (Lorr Scale) and Treatment Outcome: Psychotherapy Patients

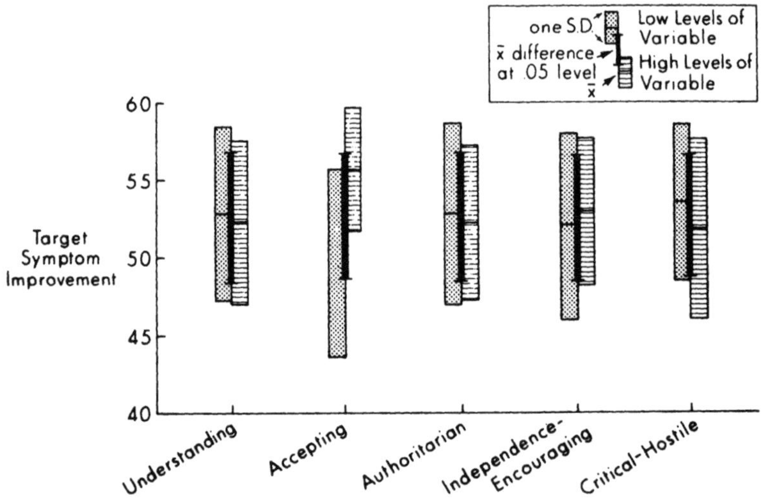


The second section of the questionnaire asked for the patient's comments on his or her expectations of therapy and how well these expectations were met. The questions were open-ended and permitted a detailed response. This section included a question about the effects of the four-month time limit. No real pattern emerged from these responses. Several patients of both therapies praised the personalities of their therapists. Several of the successful behavior therapy patients reported initial expectations of an analytic type of therapy, but were able to adjust to the technical differences of approach. All of the behavior therapy failures reported having encountered therapeutic goals, orientations, and relationships which were different from their expectations. This is to be ex-

Figure 56

Patient Perception of Behavior Therapist Behavior (Lorr Scale) and Treatment Outcome: Behavior Therapy Patients

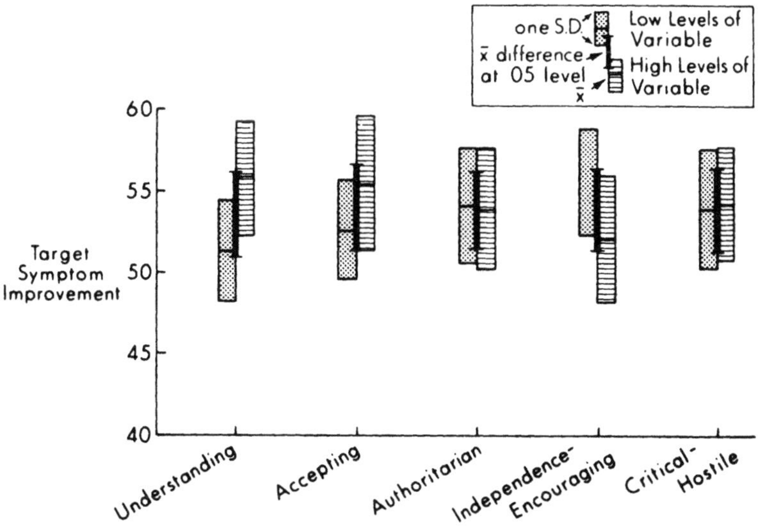


pected, since the questionnaire was answered after completion of therapy. A patient who was unable to adjust to an unexpected kind of therapy would likely be relatively unsuccessful while one who found therapy very helpful must have adjusted relatively well to it. All four of the behavior therapy failures sought further therapy with an analytically oriented therapist whose orientation presumably coincided more closely with their expectations. Three of these were pleased with the change.

Three (two psychotherapy; one behavior therapy) successful patients complained about the four-month time limit, but one found it helpful. Among treatment failures, responses to this question were more revealing. None of the behavior therapy failures complained about the briefness of therapy but four of the nine psychotherapy failures did so, three of them bitterly. Probably behavioral methods are better suited to treatment of four months' duration, so that even if it has not succeeded at four months, patients feel it has been given more of a fair trial and feel less frustrated when therapy is cut off. Possibly psychotherapists feel less comfortable with time-limited therapy and communicate their uneasiness to their patients. At any rate, short time limitations seemed more likely to frustrate patients in the context of psychotherapy than in behavior therapy.

The next section of the questionnaire consisted of thirty-two statements describing therapy, ranging from those characteristic of behavior therapy (for example, "training in muscle relaxation,") to those characteristic of psychotherapy ("explaining the relationship of your problem to early life events").They included some items characteristic of all forms of therapy regardless of theoretical orientation, for example, on the appearance and manner of the therapist. The patient rated each of these on a five-point scale from extremely important to not important.

The successful patients in both therapies placed primary importance on more or less the same items. The following items were each termed "extremely important" or "very important" by at least 70% of successful patients in both groups:

1. The personality of your doctor.
2. His helping you to understand your problems.
3. Encouraging you gradually to practice facing the things that bother you.
4. Being able to talk to an understanding person.
5. Helping you to understand yourself.

In addition, at least 70% of the successful psychotherapy patients rated as extremely or very important:

1. Encouraging you to shoulder your own responsibilities by restoring confidence in yourself.
2. The skill of your therapist.
3. His confidence that you would improve.

Nearly all these items can be classified as "encouragement, advice, or reassurance," factors common to both behavior therapy and psychotherapy.[12] None of the items regarded as very important by the majority of either group of patients describes techniques specific to one therapy. A psychotherapist might be surprised at the inclusion of "encouraging you gradually to practice facing the things that bother you" on his patients' list of important factors. Similarly a behavior therapist might be surprised that in the eyes of his successful patients most of the factors important to his success involve the patient-therapist relationship. Most noticeable is the great overlap between the two groups, suggesting that, at least from the patients' point of view, the effectiveness of treatment was due to factors common to both therapies rather than to any particular theoretical orientation or techniques.

This is consonant with the results of a study by Ryan and Gizynski,[13] in which they interviewed fourteen behavior therapy patients, most of whom had been successfully treated. In a more or less impressionistic account of these interviews, they report that the behavior modification techniques themselves were not salient to these patients. They rarely mentioned the techniques spontaneously and seemed to attach little importance to them, but they "hardly stopped talking about issues in the relationship between themselves and their therapists." However, patients may not be the best judges of what helped them, nor necessarily are they even aware of the specific techniques used by their therapists. Warmth and understanding on the part of the therapist are likely to make therapy a more pleasant experience but they may not be crucial to improvement. Certainly retrospective reports of how treatment went are heavily influenced by how the patient feels about the therapist. If the therapy has gone well the patient is more likely to consider his therapist warm and understanding, just as therapists tend to see good traits in patients who are eager to seek and accept psychiatric help.

The last section of the questionnaire asked what the patient learned in treatment about various aspects of his life. Answers to these questions seemed to fall into two categories: I, statements describing learning about past events, maladaptive feelings, and behaviors; and II, descriptions of constructive actions which require performance in the present. As an example of the first, a patient said he learned that he had been a selfish person and that people didn't really like him because of this behavior, but he offered no comments on what he could do about it. Exemplifying the second category is the patient who said he learned he must always be genuine, honest, and himself. Counting the number of statements in each of these two categories, we found that insight therapy patients made twice as many Category I as Category II statements, while behavior therapy patients made twice as many in Category II as in Category I.

This result is consistent with the theories on which the two therapies are based. Behavior therapies stress the replacement of maladaptive responses with new and different responses, while insight therapy emphasizes the importance of the patient's learning how past events are influencing current feelings and behavior patterns.

## CONCLUSIONS

Patient characteristics were related to outcome to compare the success of the three methods in changing patients with differing personality, pathology, and demographic characteristics.

*Psychotherapy: Patient Variables*

With psychotherapy the results confirmed clinical traditions. There was considerable support for the YAVIS syndrome of Schofield, who considered that young, attractive, verbal, intelligent, and successful patients did best in psychotherapy.[14] Patients who were more attractive (considered more likable by the therapist), more verbal (spoke more during therapy and in longer speech units, and gave faster reaction times when they spoke), and more "successful" (higher income, less clinical pathology), all showed most improvement. There was also a tendency for younger and more intelligent patients to improve more, despite the limited range of age and intelligence in the sample.

Differential response to psychotherapy appeared more related to broad clinical syndromes than to specific personality characteristics or symptomatology. The psychotherapists were most successful with patients who showed less overall pathology on the MMPI. This tendency for better adjusted patients to show greater improvement is consistent with several studies summarized by Luborsky *et al.*, who concluded that "Initially sicker patients do not improve as much with psychotherapy as the initially healthy do."[15] This is reminiscent of the old parable that unto every one which hath shall be given, and from him that hath not, even that he hath shall be taken away from him. The level of initial disturbance as assessed by the neuroticism scale of the EPI, the assessor ratings of target symptom severity, and work and social adjustment were unrelated to degree of improvement. However, least improvement was shown by patients with both high overall pathology on the MMPI and more severe target symptoms. In a sense these patients were doubly damned, and received significantly less help from therapy.

Our psychotherapists were less successful with patients who

showed the acting-out syndrome on the MMPI than with those who did not. While there is evidence that psychotherapy can be effective with an antisocial delinquent population[16] there is little available data as to its relative effectiveness with such a population compared to a neurotic one. Our findings, in fact, support the popular clinical assumption that traditional psychotherapy is more effective with neurotic patients whose symptoms are egodystonic than with those who act out their problems.

There was no support for the hypothesis that patients with disturbed emotions, either depression or anxiety, would show greater improvement. Despite the fairly consistent reports of greater therapeutic success associated with high scores on the depression scale of the MMPI,[17, 18, 19] there was a strong tendency in the present study for more improvement by patients who were *lowest* on the depression scale. Anxiety, as assessed by the Taylor Manifest Anxiety Scale or by its presence as one of the target symptoms, did not appear related to outcome.

None of the personality variables of the Eysenck Personality Inventory, or those of the California Psychological Inventory used in the study, appeared to discriminate between successful and unsuccessful outcome; nor did any specific symptoms.

### *Behavior Therapy: Patient Variables*

For behavior therapy there were fewer prognostic indicators. Differences in outcome for each patient variable tended to be smaller, and fewer were statistically reliable. No personality characteristics, specific symptomatology, demographic characteristics, or level of pathology were significantly related to successful outcome in behavior therapy. There were too few patients with specific phobias to investigate hypotheses concerning this syndrome. However, the more introverted or more anxious patients were *not* most responsive to behavior therapy.

In fact, the opposite was found. The most acting-out patients (as judged by the MMPI) tended to show the most improvement. This suggests that disorders of behavior are amenable to treatment by behavior therapy.

*Wait-List Variables*

There were no specific problems that showed more "spontaneous" improvement in wait-list patients. There was a slight tendency for those with less overall pathology on the MMPI to improve more. Although no MMPI differences were statistically reliable, high scoring patients on all clinical scales except the depression scale averaged less improvement than low scoring patients. The amount of improvement was independent of the other measures used.

*Psychotherapy: Patient-Therapist Relationship*

The quality of the relationship between patient and therapist appeared critical for success in psychoanalytically oriented therapy. Patients liked by their therapists improved considerably more than those who were less liked. Other studies do not consistently support this finding, despite its intuitive appeal. A multitude of factors can of course enter into a global judgment of liking—including both personal attraction and "good" therapy behavior by the patient. Nevertheless, it would seem plausible that a better therapeutic relationship is more likely to be formed with someone whom you like than with someone you do not. There was also a strong tendency for patients who improved more to perceive their therapists as "warm" and "genuine" persons. The question remains whether certain techniques produce good therapy behavior from the patient or whether the behavior of a good patient results in a different type of therapist behavior. Does developing attraction for the patient provide an atmosphere which allows the patient to verbalize his feelings more completely? Or do patients who are able to discuss their problems more completely become more likable?

Interpersonal attraction and its resultant interaction is not simply defined by levels of accurate empathy, depth of interpersonal contact, therapist self-congruence, or unconditional positive regard offered by the therapist. Ratings of these factors from the fifth interview were unrelated to outcome. The lack of predictive power may have resulted from the relatively high levels of these factors offered by all the therapists in this study. As Strupp and Bergin suggest, "It seems more reasonable to conclude that once the therapist has achieved a fair level of therapeutic skills and is successful in providing a modicum of warmth, empathy, and so on, outcome is more importantly a function of technical competence and patient characteristics."[20] Experienced therapists may thus be able to offer sufficiently high levels of these factors regardless of their personal attitude toward the patient. Their positive feeling for the patient, or lack of it, may have its effect elsewhere in the treatment process. Moreover these variables may have less relevance to non-client-centered treatments. There were marked differences in speech between successful and less successful patients. Successful patients took up a greater proportion of the therapeutic hour with their talk. This was not because they spoke more often, but because they spoke for a longer time when they did speak and responded more quickly to the therapist's comments. These findings exactly duplicate the results of a previous study with less experienced therapists.[21] They demonstrate the potential of such conceptually simple objective measures of the process of therapy.

In general, analysis of the techniques of the psychoanalytically oriented therapists provided a picture similar to the one they hold of themselves.

*Behavior Therapy: Patient-Therapist Relationships*

For behavior therapy, the measures we used did not discriminate well between successful and unsuccessful treatment. Some trends were evident but these tended not to be statistically reliable. The only major significant variable was the duration of the patient's speech. Again, successful patients used longer statements. This factor was predictive in both therapies. The other measures showed clear differences between the two treatments, but with little relationship to outcome.

*The Two Therapies Compared*

Thus the treatments were both by definition and practice different. Two groups of therapists did different things in treatment, yet they seemed to achieve basically similar results. We were successful in identifying some patient characteristics and process variables which were related to successful outcome for psychotherapy, less so for behavior therapy. This may mean that psychotherapy is more dependent than behavior therapy upon matching the right combination of patient characteristics and therapeutic techniques. Or it may mean that we happened to select measures that relate to success in psychotherapy but not behavior therapy. The first alternative appears more likely since the results of psychotherapy were more variable: more patients showed greater improvement and more showed less improvement than in behavior therapy. The mean improvement (T) scores were similar, but the variance for psychotherapy was significantly greater ($F = 2.227$; $p < .05$).

Behavior therapy, instead of being limited to patients with circumscribed problems such as phobias, may in fact be suitable for a wider range of patients than traditional psychotherapy. Analytically oriented therapy as practiced in this study seemed to work best with a certain type of patient. In contrast, a broader range of problems was susceptible to the behavioral techniques used. Given the right combination of patient and therapist, psychotherapy was as effective, or more effective, than behavior therapy. With the wrong combination it was less effective.

There are many possible explanations for this finding. Frank believes that any therapy merely accelerates spontaneous improvement. Behavioral techniques then may simply work more quickly to accentuate this improvement in a greater variety of patients. Alternatively, focused behavioral techniques may be more effective in producing modest yet consistent gains than the more diffuse techniques of insight therapy.

Finally, behavior therapy may have available a wider range of techniques to meet the various needs of various patients. For example, in addition to standard behavioral techniques, such as desensitization and assertive training, behavior therapists used virtually the same number of interpretive statements as did psychotherapists. Although these interpretations were qualitatively different from those of psychotherapists, they served the same purpose of providing a rationale of causality along theoretical lines. This suggests that behavior therapists may have had more options available to them. However, the majority of successful psychotherapy patients reported that one of the most useful aspects of their treatment was "the therapist encouraging you to practice facing things that bother you." This is reminiscent of some form of desensitization and was certainly not one of the professed techniques, either in our stipulative definitions or in the psychotherapists' own accounts of therapy. It is at least plausible that the psychotherapists used some behavior strategies.

# 8 Summary

One hundred twenty-six people applying for psychotherapy at a university psychiatric outpatient clinic were interviewed at length by an experienced psychiatrist, and ninety-four, suffering from moderately severe neuroses and personality disorders, were accepted for treatment in this study. We excluded those who were considered too disturbed to be assigned to a four-month wait-list control group, those whose disturbance seemed so minor that therapy was not indicated, and those who seemed more likely to respond to some other treatment (for example, antidepressant medication) than to any kind of psychotherapy. In the course of the assessment interview, the patients were rated for severity of illness on many different scales, and they also completed the Eysenck, Minnesota Multiphasic Personality, and California Psychological Inventories together with the Mill Hill Vocabulary Scale.

There were two principal measures of psychological change. One, the Structured and Scaled Interview to Assess Maladjustment (SSIAM), yielded estimates of work maladjustment and of social maladjustment. The other was the assessor's rating of the severity of the patient's target symptoms, the three most important specific difficulties that had led him to seek therapy, and from which he most desired relief. Thus, there was a standard measure of general adjustment, and a measure of the specific problems of the individual patient.

At the same time, a research assistant interviewed a close friend or relative of the patient (the "informant") who also made ratings of the patient's work and social adjustment.

The patients were assigned without their assessors' knowledge to the wait list, to a behavior therapist, or to an analytically oriented psychotherapist. The assignment was random except that the treatment groups were equalized as to the sex of the patient and according to a rough measure of pathology (higher versus lower scores on the neuroticism scale of the Eysenck Personality Inventory).

The control patients were promised therapy in four months' time; they were given their assessor's telephone number to call in case of a crisis; and were telephoned several times during the four month waiting period by a research assistant who asked how they were getting on and assured them they would soon be assigned a therapist. They thus received most of the nonspecific aspects of therapy: a long initial interview, the promise of help and expectation of improvement, access to crisis help, and a continuing (though very brief, superficial, and not intentionally therapeutic) relationship with an interested person.

The other patients were assigned to one of three experienced psychoanalytically oriented therapists or to one of three experienced behavior therapists, who treated them for four months (an average of about fourteen sessions). Behavior therapists emphasized techniques of behavior modification, such as systematic desensitization and assertive training, but did not entirely exclude discussion of feelings. Psychoanalytically oriented therapists emphasized insight into feelings and the quality of the therapeutic relationship itself. Two of the psychotherapists were psychoanalysts, and the third was in personal analysis with a training analyst. With a few exceptions for technical reasons, each patient's fifth therapy session was tape recorded. Patients paid for therapy through the outpatient clinic on its usual sliding scale based on income. After the first therapy session, the therapist rated the patient's work and social adjustment on a scale like that used by the patient, the assessor, and the informant.

Four months after the initial interview each patient was interviewed again by his original assessor, and both again rated the severity of each target symptom, so that symptomatic improvement could be determined by comparing the rating of a symptom's severity after four months with the rating of its initial severity. The SSIAM was again administered, and amount of change on its work and social scales were similarly calculated. The assessor was not told what treatment any patient had received, but his ratings were not entirely "blind," as several patients spontaneously referred to their therapy during the assessment interview. Before this interview, the assessor refreshed his memory of the patient by rereading his original case report, but he did not look at his initial numerical ratings of the patient.

Only sixty-five informants could be interviewed at this time. They again estimated patients' social, work, and sexual adjustment, and similar change scores were calculated here. Therapists also repeated their ratings of their patients' work, social, and sexual adjustments after four months of therapy.

At this time eleven of the control patients no longer desired to be assigned to a therapist. The others were placed in treatment with senior residents who were mostly of a psychoanalytical orientation. Nine psychotherapy patients and fifteen behavior therapy patients also received varying amounts of additional treatment, in most cases from their original therapists. This made it difficult to evaluate results from further follow-up interviews, which were held one year and two years after original assessment.

## RESULTS

At four months, all three groups had improved significantly on the severity of their target symptoms. Both treated groups of patients had improved significantly more than the wait-list group, but there was no significant difference in the amount of improvement between the psychotherapy and the behavior therapy groups. On the work scale of the SSIAM behavior therapy patients had improved significantly, while psychotherapy and wait-list patients showed only marginal improvement. Likewise on the SSIAM social scale, only the behavior therapy and wait-list patients improved significantly. However there was no significant difference in *amount* of improvement between the three groups either for work or social adjustment. On a rating scale of overall improvement, 93% of the behavior therapy patients contrasted to 77% of the psychotherapy and wait-list patients were considered either improved or recovered ($\chi^2 = 3.93$; $p < .05$).

At this time there was no significant effect on improvement due to the sex of the patient, the severity of neuroticism (as measured by the Eysenck Personality Inventory), or the amount of the therapist's experience. However, all therapists had considerable experience.

At the one-year follow-up, improvement was maintained or continued in most patients. The behavior therapy group was still significantly improved on target symptoms and work and social adjustment. The psychotherapy group was now also significantly improved on all three measures, having continued to improve their social adjustment in the eight-month interim. The wait-list patients were no longer significantly improved in work adjustment but were still improved in target symptoms and social adjustment. The only significant intergroup difference at one year was that the behavior therapy patients were still significantly more improved on target symptom severity than the control patients.

It is difficult to evaluate these one-year results since so many members of each group had different therapeutic experiences after the initial four months. If, instead, we compare only patients who had no therapy after four months, the results were substantially similar. All groups maintained significant symptomatic improvement; behavior therapy and psychotherapy patients were significantly improved in work adjustment but wait-list patients only marginally so. Psychotherapy patients were significantly improved in social adjustment while behavior therapy and wait-list patients showed only marginal change. However, the groups did not differ significantly on amount of improvement for any measure. These results must also be cautiously interpreted: they were not confounded by intervening therapy but we cannot know the effect of the subjects' self-selection. However, we do know that these patients who decided against further therapy (or against *any* therapy, in the case of the control patients) were no different from the other patients on any psychological or demographic dimension we measured. Specifically, they were not patients who all were "cured" in four months' therapy and needed no more; nor were they patients for all of whom therapy was such a failure that they were not inclined to seek more.

There was no evidence of any symptom substitution in any group. On the contrary, patients whose target symptoms improved often reported improvement in other, less important symptoms as well.

At the two-year follow-up of sixty-one patients—all who could be interviewed at that time—the great majority in all groups had increased or maintained significant improvement both on symptomatic and adjustment measures and on the MMPI scales. Unfortunately, the psychotherapy patients who could be reassessed at two years proved to be those who had already shown most improvement at one year. Because of this sample bias, a comparison with the behavior therapy and wait-list patients, who were representative of their original samples, was not feasible. However, the results do indicate that the initial improvement was not a transitory phenomenon, and was maintained by most patients without further supportive therapy between the one- and two-year assessments.

## PROCESS VARIABLES AND OUTCOME

Four four-minute samples of each fifth taped therapy session were rated on the Truax variables and on the Lennard and Bernstein categories by two experienced raters. On the Truax dimensions, behavior therapists were rated as providing significantly higher levels of accurate empathy and self-congruence and a significantly greater degree of interpersonal contact than the psychotherapists. Levels of warmth, or unconditional positive regard, were not significantly different between groups. Truax's variables are predictive of success in some (especially client-centered) therapeutic studies but in this study none of them were correlated with the degree of patient improvement. But it is nevertheless interesting that behavior therapists, who are often thought of as providing a cold, mechanical, unfeeling, and superficial service, are rated as providing equal or higher levels of all these interpersonal process measures.

The Lennard and Bernstein ratings showed that the topic discussed was more often initiated by the patient in psychotherapy and by the therapist in behavior therapy. This is consistent with the common belief that behavior therapists are more directive of the course of treatment than are psychotherapists. None of the Lennard and Bernstein categories was significantly related to improvement on target symptoms, indicating that this difference in style may be simply that, with no important effect on the outcome of therapy.

An analysis of speech patterns—who spends how much time talking—in recordings of whole therapy sessions indicated that while behavior therapists and their patients spent roughly equal amounts of time talking, psychotherapy patients talked about three times as much as their therapists. While behavior therapists talked twice as much as psychotherapists did, not surprisingly psychotherapy patients talked twice as much as behavior therapy patients. This too characterizes behavior therapists' greater control over and direct participation in the therapy. In both psychotherapy and behavior therapy, patients who spoke in longer utterances improved significantly more on their target symptoms than patients who spoke in short utterances. In psychotherapy those patients who talked more altogether improved significantly more, but this was not true for behavior therapy.

Each statement made by a therapist in every patient's fifth therapeutic session was classified by two reliable raters as belonging to one of the following seven categories: questions, giving information, clarification and interpretation, nondirective statements, directive statements, approval, and disapproval. There were two significant differences between behavior therapists and psychotherapists. First, behavior therapists made more statements giving information not directly related to the patient's problem. This reflects their greater readiness to answer patients' questions directly, where psychotherapists tend to reflect such questions. Second, behavior therapists used more statements in the imperative mode, directing the patient to do something. This also is in keeping with the general impression that behavior therapists are more directive than psychotherapists. In the psychotherapy group, patients receiving fewer "clarification and interpretation" statements improved significantly more than those receiving many, but this paradoxical result did not hold true for the behavior therapy patients.

## PATIENT AND RELATIONSHIP CHARACTERISTICS AND OUTCOME

There are interesting differences in the types of patients who responded to psychotherapy and to behavior therapy. Using a composite rating of target symptom change as the criterion of improvement, we found that, in psychotherapy, patients with more severe pathology (as measured on the MMPI) improved less on their target symptoms than did initially relatively healthier patients. This difference was especially clear for the hysteria and psychopathic deviate scales, which often indicate antisocial acting-out behavior. For behavior therapy patients, on the other hand, the amount of improvement was much less affected by the general level of pathology as measured by the MMPI. Furthermore, what consistent effect there was suggested that behavior therapy patients with *more* initial pathology on acting-out scales (hysteria and mania) improved more than initially less disturbed patients. In keeping with this, there was a consistent tendency for patients with relatively greater pathology on those MMPI scales that suggest acting-out behavior to improve more with behavior therapy than with psychotherapy. (However, this was significant only in the case of hysteria.) Similar results, though not nearly so consistent, appeared on the California and Eysenck Personality Inventories. There was some tendency for psychotherapy patients with higher self-acceptance, greater self-control and sociability, and less (EPI) neuroticism to show more symptomatic improvement than did more disturbed patients; there was no such tendency for behavior therapy patients.

The effects of demographic variables on outcome did not reach statistical significance but were very consistent. Relatively greater success in psychotherapy was associated with greater youth, higher intelligence, higher income, being female, being married, coming from a smaller family, and being not the first-born. These factors seemed to have no effect on the outcome of behavior therapy.

There were some differences in outcome of both psychotherapy and behavior therapy related to both the patients' and therapists' perceptions of their relationship. Psychotherapy patients improved more who were more liked by their therapists, who were rated as resembling their therapists' usual patients, and who were considered "suitable" for this treatment. These factors apparently have no effect on the outcome of behavior therapy patients, but there was a tendency for the latter to improve more if their therapists felt comfortable with them and found them interesting. For both psychotherapy and behavior therapy groups, there was a strong tendency for patients who reported greater nonpossessive warmth, genuineness, and accurate empathy to show more improvement. This provides some evidence that the patient-therapist relationship is important in both treatments, but these data must be interpreted cautiously. Both patient and therapist ratings were made at the end of therapy; and a therapist might be as likely to like a patient because the patient improved, as the patient might be to improve as an indirect result of the therapist's liking him.

## CONCLUSIONS

First, it is remarkable that all three groups of patients significantly improved in four months. The control group was by no means "untreated," but it improved considerably without any formal therapy. Nevertheless, both groups of formally treated patients improved significantly more than the control patients on their target symptoms. This is rather clear evidence that therapy in general "works," that the improvement of patients in therapy is not entirely due either to "spontaneous recovery," or to the placebo effect of the nonspecific aspects of therapy, such as arousal of hope, expectation of help, and an initial cathartic interview. Our control patients were exposed to all these nonspecific aspects and yet improved significantly less than treated patients.

Second, behavior therapy is at least as effective, and possibly more so than psychotherapy with the sort of moderately severe neuroses and personality disorders that are typical of clinic populations. This should help to dispel the impression that behavior therapy is useful only with phobias and restricted "unitary" problems. In fact, only the behavior therapy group in this study had improved significantly on both the work and the social measures of general adjustment at four months. Behavior therapy is clearly a *generally* useful treatment.

Third, there is evidence that behavior therapy can effectively deal with a broader range of patients than can psychotherapy. Both treatments are apparently effective with the classical stereotype of the good patient: a verbal, intelligent, well-educated young woman of reasonably high income, who is less severely disturbed to begin with, and whose disorder tends toward neurosis and introversion rather than personality disorders or any kind of acting-out behavior. In this study, psychotherapists had more success with patients like this than with those with opposite characteristics, whereas these differences seemed not to matter to behavior therapists. The latter tended to achieve more symptomatic improvement with disturbed, acting-out patients than the psychotherapists did.

Fourth, it is clear that behavior therapists and psychotherapists provided distinctive treatments. We were impressed by the similarity among therapists in each group. While theoretical differences between the senior and the second behavior therapist had begun at the time of this study, their behavior in therapy was much closer to that of each other than to any of the psychotherapists. Differences between behavior therapists and psychotherapists were evident not only in their formulations of their patients' problems and in their clinical strategies, but also in their pattern of interaction with patients. Behavior therapists were more active than psychotherapists; they more frequently gave explicit advice and instructions, provided information, presented their own value judgments, controlled the content of the conversation, dominated the conversation verbally, and achieved a deeper level of interpersonal contact and empathy than did the more passive psychotherapists. Behavior therapists were seen by the patients as more genuine persons but also as encouraging less independence than the psychotherapists.

Fifth, the patient-therapist relationship appears to be a critical factor in the success of psychotherapy, and important in behavior therapy as well. In psychotherapy, but not behavior therapy, patients who were liked by their therapists showed greater improvement than those who were less liked. Although Truax variables rated from therapy sessions were unrelated to outcome, patients in both groups who themselves reported higher levels of warmth, empathy, or genuineness in their therapists tended to show greater improvement. Successful patients in both therapies rated the personal interaction with the therapist as the single most important part of their treatment.

Finally, these data provide evidence that therapy of both kinds is effective. They do not show that behavior therapy is more effective than psychotherapy, but they do clearly indicate that behavior therapy is not only useful for the typical outpatient population of mixed neurotics, but equally effective in providing symptomatic relief and in improving the patient's ability to cope with life.

# APPENDICES
# NOTES
# INDEX

# APPENDIX 1

# STRUCTURED AND SCALED INTERVIEW TO ASSESS MALADJUSTMENT (SSIAM)

The words summarize the questionnaire's main features.

*Structured.* The interview is structured by an orderly series of questions which encourage the patient to describe different facets of his adjustment. The interviewer may paraphrase the questions to clarify their meaning and may discuss both the questions and answers before making a rating. This conversational style avoids the impression of encountering an impersonal clerk charged with the task of completing a form. Rather, it maintains the atmosphere of consulting with a doctor who is trying to understand the salient features of a patient's life.

The questions ask the patient to describe his behavior and reactions in five different social contexts. These are work-school, social-leisure, family, marriage, and sex. Within each context there are five questions that deal with behavior, one with interpersonal friction, and three with distress. For example, in the field of work the questions that deal with behavior are: "Do you have difficulty in holding down a job?" "How well do you do your work?" "Are you making progress in your career?" "Are you working too hard?" "Are you able to stand up for yourself at work?" The question about friction with other people is: "Do you tend to have quarrels and ill-feelings with people at work?" The questions about subjective distress are: "Do you find your work interesting?" "Do you feel upset or uncomfortable or worried at work for any reason?" "Do you feel inferior at work?" This structured interview allows the same questions to be put in the same order to a series of patients, or to an individual patient at different times, or to another person who is able to give independent information about the patient.

*Scaled.* The information gained by this structured interviewing can be rated quickly on prepared scales. Three examples of the scales are shown in Table A-1 and are discussed at the end of this Appendix. For each question there is a corresponding scale on which the interviewer rates the information about that particular aspect of the patient's adjustment. A scale consists of a vertical line with scale points, five of which are identified by anchoring definitions. During the construction of the scales, each set of definitions was reworded frequently until four consultant psychotherapists reached agreement that the lowest definition represents adjustment which requires no treatment, and the highest definition describes the most serious maladjustment likely to be encountered in psychoneurotic outpatients. The three intermediate definitions represent about equal steps of maladjustment between those extremes.

To avoid unrealistic ratings, the interviewer may rate the answer to a question as "not known" or "not applicable." To facilitate consistent use of the scales, a number of operational definitions and instructions are provided to guide the rater.

*Interview.* The tone of the questions and discussion resembles a clinical interview. The topics progress comfortably from the public and familiar aspects of a patient's life which he is used to talking about, such as the number of jobs he has held in the last four months, toward the more personal and private aspects of his life which he is not used to discussing, such as his sexual adjustment. The wording of the questions is simple, direct, and tactful. Discussion flows easily from one question to the next. After covering the last area, sex, the interviewer asks some overall questions which help to bring the interview to its natural conclusion.

*Assess.* The SSIAM not only gives the interview structure, but permits information to be measured. The rating on each scale gives an item score. Item scores may be added to give raw scores for the different social areas or types of items, or used to yield scores derived from a factor analysis. Six factors were found in a study of 164 adults who were acceptable for outpatient psychotherapy.* The factors were: social isolation, work inadequacy, friction with family, dependence on family, social dissatisfaction, and friction outside the family. Scores may be based on data from the patient himself or from a close relative or friend. These factors are relatively independent and show a high degree of interrater agreement.

*Maladjustment.* The interview is directed toward finding evidence of maladjustment rather than of adjustment. The interviewer thus maintains a constant set of looking for pathology. A constant set helps to standardize assessment because the interest of assessors may vary with the context. When assessing patients for the first time, the set of the diagnostician is often toward finding pathology. In assessing after treatment, the therapist may be inclined to notice evidence of improvement. The SSIAM is designed to help a rater maintain a consistent set toward obtaining evidence of maladjustment. In case of doubt between one level of rating and another, the

*B.J. Gurland, N.J. Yorkston, K. Goldberg, J.L. Fliess, R.B. Sloane, and A.H. Cristol. "The structured and scaled interview to assess maladjustment (SSIAM). II. Factor analysis, reliability, and validity." *Archives of General Psychiatry* 27: 264-267, 1972.

interviewer decides in favor of maladjustment rather than adjustment. No attempt is made to assess the patient's symptoms, personality, physical health, or mental state. For example, there are no assessments of autonomic symptoms, depression, or hallucinations or thought disorder. The SSIAM is used to assess social maladjustment independently from psychiatric or medical diagnosis.

*Examples in Table A-1*

The first item is W4 from the work pathology scale. This attempts to measure how efficiently the patient uses his work time. Q at the top of the page is the question asked the patient,

TABLE A-1. Examples of SSIAM Scales

| W4 Over-Working | S4 Apathetic in Leisure | M6 Friction |
|---|---|---|
| Q: Do you work too hard? (e.g. do you rush, try to do too much, miss your coffee, tea or lunch breaks, work excess overtime even weekends?) | Q: Do you have any particular spare-time interests and activities? | Q: Is there any tension, coolness or outright quarreling in your marital family? |
| 1) Include perfectionistic overwork.<br>2) 'Other areas of life' include vacations, weekends, social leisure activities, family life.<br>3) 'Personal time': justifiable time off work, e.g. for dentistry or personal business. | 1) A 'developed interest' is a growing knowledge of, and strong preference for an activity (e.g. sports, gardening, or reading). | 1) Disregard whether others are responsible (but rate in #M10E)<br>2) Include differences of opinion over sex, responsibilities and authority. |
| Working time completely crowds out 'other areas of life.' | No involvement in spare time interests. | Marriage breaking up. Gross incompatibility. |
| Working time intrudes markedly into 'other areas of life.' | Does passively what others do (watches TV *only* if others suggest it). | Violence or marked estrangement or radical differences of opinion. |
| Work confined to reasonable hours, but rushed and crowded. | Has interests but they are 'underdeveloped' and undiscriminating (watches anything on TV). | Quite frequent quarrels or coolness or chronic differences of opinion. |
| Work pace and duration reasonable but never feels free to take 'personal time' off. | Has preferences for certain interests but not well 'developed'. | Some excessive tensions or misunderstandings or disagreements. |
| Puts in no more than a reasonable day's work and takes 'personal time' off when necessary. | Fairly well developed interests (sports, gardening). | Reasonably smooth and warm relationship. |
| __Not known | __Not known | __Not known |
| __Not applicable | __Not applicable | __Not applicable |

"Do you work too hard?" Besides the elaboration in the question: "do you rush?" etc., the numbered points dealing with perfectionistic overwork, definitions or other areas of life and personal time are intended to clarify the question for the rater. Then a scale follows with eleven check points, five with anchoring definitions. These five are shown in the table.

After consultation with the patient, the rater marks the check point which most closely represents the patient's condition. For scoring, these points are given numerical values. The top check point represents greatest pathology and is rated 10. The bottom check point, if it applies, is rated 0 and represents least pathology. Intermediate points are given intermediate values, so that a single number can represent the patient's condition in respect to each question. The five anchoring definitions are opposite points 1, 3, 5, 7, and 9.

Questions S4 and M6 on use of leisure time and friction with others are similarly shown. The first comes from the social-leisure scale and the second from the marriage scale.

# APPENDIX 2
# METHOD OF RANDOM ASSIGNMENT TO GROUPS

The assignment procedure was carrried out by drawing up four lists of empty slots—18 slots in the male high-pathology list, 18 slots in the male low-pathology list, 27 slots in the female high-pathology list, and 27 slots in the female low-pathology list. Each of the 9 treatment subgroups (for example, behavior therapist 3, or wait-list group 1) was given a number, and a random-number table was used to assign the name of a subgroup to each empty slot. Each subgroup occupied 2 slots on each of the 2 male lists. For example, 2 high-pathology males and 2 low-pathology males would be assigned to each of the 6 therapists and each of the 3 wait-list subgroups. Similarly, each subgroup occupied 3 slots on each of the 2 female lists (i.e., 3 high-pathology females and 3 low-pathology females would be assigned to each of the 9 subgroups).

As an example, the first female low-pathology patient accepted into the study would be assigned to the subgroup which had thus randomly been assigned to fill the first slot on the female low-pathology list. It was therefore known before any patients were interviewed that, say, the first low-pathology female accepted would be assigned to Wait-List Subgroup 1; the second low-pathology female accepted would be assigned to Wait-List Subgroup 3; the third to Behavior Therapist 3; the fourth to Psychotherapist 2, and so until 27 low-pathology females had been accepted into the study and assigned to subgroups.

While the patient was being assessed, the research assistant could score his Eysenck Personality Inventory, consult the list appropriate to his sex and pathology level, and assign him to the subgroup occupying the next available slot on that list. If the assessor accepted the patient, the research assistant could then immediately either tell the patient that he was on the wait list (with accompanying explanation) or give him the name and telephone number of the therapist who would be expecting his call. The assessor was not told to what subgroup his patient had been assigned.

APPENDIX 3

# STIPULATIVE DEFINITIONS OF PSYCHOTHERAPY AND BEHAVIOR THERAPY

**A. Elements in common**

There is a therapist who:

1. Is available to spend specified times with the patient
2. Shows an interest
3. Takes a biographical psychiatric history
4. Formulates the patient's problems
5. Attempts to reconstruct possible original causes of the disorder
6. Looks for continuing causes of the difficulty
7. Aims to produce a change which benefits the patient. The aims may include:
   a. removing or reducing subjective complaints
   b. removing or reducing recurrent behavior which disturbs the patient or other people
   c. promoting better patterns of behavior
8. Corrects misconceptions
9. Elucidates objectives
10. Answers questions
11. Uses few technical terms
12. May use abreaction in some instances
13. Discusses, on its merits, any criticism of the rationale and methods of treatment

14. Sometimes uses direct suggestion, for example may say that the patient will feel better without offering supportive evidence (but does not employ repeated suggestions as used in hypnosis)
15. May attempt to change family, employer, or doctor

**B. Excluded from both psychotherapy and behavior therapy**

Both therapies will be undertaken without use of regular medication. Ideally, no medication at all will be used, but drugs may be prescribed for use in acute circumstances. If drugs are used, sedatives at night will be prescribed rather than tranquilizers by day. As a rule, however, drugs of psychiatric importance will not be employed.

Carbon dioxide inhalation and injections of methohexitone may be used in treatment sessions by the behavior therapy group.

If any medication is employed, the therapist will note the dosage and period of time over which it is employed.

**C. Items characteristic of (b) behavior therapy and (p) psychotherapy**

1. Specific advice
   b) Given frequently
   p) Given infrequently
2. Transference interpretation
   b) Avoided
   p) May be given
3. Interpretation of resistance
   b) Not used
   p) Used
4. Dreams
   b) Polite lack of interest: not used in treatment

p) Interest in reported dreams which may be used in treatment

5. Level of anxiety
   b) Diminished when possible except in implosive therapy
   p) Maintain some anxiety as long as it does not disrupt behavior
6. Training in relaxation
   b) Directly undertaken
   p) Only an indirect consequence of sitting, and perhaps the example of the therapist
7. Desensitization
   b) Directly undertaken
   p) Only an indirect consequence of talking in comfortable circumstances with uncritical therapist
8. Practical retraining
   b) Directly undertaken
   p) Not emphasized
9. Training in appropriately assertive action
   b) Directly undertaken and encouraged in everyday life
   p) Only indirectly encouraged in everyday life
   Assertive or aggressive speech which would be inappropriate in everyday life permitted in therapeutic session.
10. Symptoms
    b) Interest in the report of symptoms, may explain biologically
    p) Report of symptoms discouraged, may interpret symbolically
11. Childhood memories
    b) Usually history-taking only
    p) Usually further memories looked for
12. Aversion, e.g. electric shock
    b) May be used
    p) Not used

13. Observers of treatment session
    b) May be permitted
    p) Not usually permitted
14. Deliberate attempts to stop behavior such as thoughts which make the patient anxious
    b) May be used
    p) Rarely directly attempted
15. Role training
    b) May be used
    p) Not used
16. Repetition of motor habits
    b) May be used
    p) Not used

# APPENDIX 4

# TWO-TAILED AND ONE-TAILED *t* TESTS

There is some controversy in the statistical literature concerning the appropriateness of "two-tailed" versus "one-tailed" tests of significance. If a one-tailed test is used, the prediction is tested that change will be shown in one direction only. For example, in the present study one might predict that all patients will improve. With a two-tailed test, the significance of change in either direction is tested, i.e. that patients may improve or become worse. A two-tailed test is less likely to show significant improvement than a one-tailed test at a given level of significance, since it examines both ends of the distribution of change scores. In the present study, two-tailed tests have been used in testing for within-group differences between initial and post-therapy assessments, as well as for between-group comparisons, on the assumption that certain subgroups of patients may become worse on certain measures. In fact they do worsen on certain measures, and it is worthwhile to test the significance of such change.

However, some readers may feel that the principal question is whether or not groups improve and that one-tailed tests would be more appropriate. Therefore we will report as "marginally" significant all within-group comparisons of initial versus post-treatment status which are statistically significant at the .05 level for a one-tailed test but only .10 significant for a two-tailed test. In this way readers whose assumptions differ may draw their own conclusions.

# APPENDIX 5
# LENNARD AND BERNSTEIN SCALE OF THERAPIST INFORMATIONAL SPECIFICITY

Category 1 refers to statements in which the therapist indicates that he is listening passively and merely encourages the patient to continue ("I see" and "um-hm"). Such comments encourage the patient to talk further without limiting him in any way, and provide no information that the patient can use to limit his choice of topics.

Statements in category 2 indicate that the therapist is listening and actively encourages the patient to continue. The main difference between categories 1 and 2 is that the therapist is more active in category 2.

In category 3 the patient is limited to one topic area, but within that topic he can select from a range of information available to him. Statements in this category indicate some control over the content of the interaction because the patient is limited to a single, albeit broad, topic. Such statements as "How about talking about your work?" or "What did you think about the last session?" are included in this category.

In category 4 the therapist refers to a specific proposition which has already been introduced in the immediately most recent antecedent interaction. This category differs from number 3 because it limits the patient to a specific idea.

In category 5 the therapist introduces a new proposition.

This differs from category 3, in that the patient is limited to a more specific topic, and differs from category 4 because it is a new topic which the therapist takes the initiative in introducing.

Statements in category 6 introduce a sequence of new propositions, thus exerting some control over the content of most of the conversation.

Category 7 includes items which introduce specific propositions with the intention of eliciting a particular item of information, asking for specific information.

In category 8 the therapist excludes a specific topic or proposition as a subject for communication.

# APPENDIX 6

# REGRESSION TRANSFORMATION

In assessing group differences in therapeutic outcome, change scores were calculated for each patient by subtracting the severity of each target symptom at the four-month assessment from its severity at initial assessment. This procedure was justified since there were no group differences at initial assessment, and all groups in effect started at a common baseline. When many different groupings are made, as in the case of splitting groups into High and Low on the basis of each patient measure and each process factor, chances are that some of these groups would differ from one another on their status at initial assessment. The use of simple difference scores in these cases might lead to biased results. The patient whose symptoms are initially mild and is completely recovered at four months, can obviously show much less improvement on a difference score than a patient whose symptoms are initially severe and who also recovers completely. Both patients may end treatment at the same level, but a comparison of their degree of improvement would be biased in favor of the patient who started with more severe symptoms.

For this reason a single index of improvement was calculated for each patient in the following manner. The severity ratings of the three target symptoms at initial assessment and at four months were each summed. A change score was taken by using a regression transformation which effectively removes the influence of differences in baseline, and provides the single index of improvement which is independent of the initial values. The formula, used by Lacey* and others, is:

$$\Delta = \frac{z_1 - r_{01} z_0}{\sqrt{1 - r_{01}^2}}$$

where $z_1$ = four-month rating in standard score form
$z_0$ = initial rating in standard score form
$r_{01}$ = correlation between initial and four-month ratings

For easier calculation and to simplify presentation of results, these obtained delta or change measures in standard score form were further transformed into T scores with a mean of 50 and a standard deviation of 10. Scores above 50 therefore represent relatively greater improvement.

*J. I. Lacey. "The evaluation of autonomic responses: Toward a general solution," *Annals of the New York Academy of Sciences* 67: 123-164, 1956.

# NOTES

## 1. Introduction

1. R.H. Geertsma and R.J. Stoller. "The consistency of psychiatrists' clinical judgments." *Journal of Nervous and Mental Disease* 137:58-66, 1963.

2. L.C. Kolb. *Noyes' Modern Clinical Psychiatry*, 7th ed. Philadelphia: Saunders, 1968.

3. F.C. Redlich and D.X. Freedman. *The Theory and Practice of Psychiatry*. New York: Basic Books, 1966, p. 347.

4. American Psychiatric Association. *Diagnostic and Statistical Manual of Mental Disorders*, 2nd ed. Washington: American Psychiatric Association, 1968.

5. L.R. Wolberg. *The Technique of Psychotherapy*. New York: Grune and Stratton, 1954, p. 3.

6. H.H. Strupp, R.E. Fox, and K. Lessler. *Patients View Their Psychotherapy*. Baltimore: Johns Hopkins Press, 1969.

7. B.J. Gurland, N.J. Yorkston, A.R. Stone, J.D. Frank, and J.L. Fliess. "The structured and scaled interview to assess maladjustment (SSIAM). I. Description, rationale, and development." *Archives of General Psychiatry* 27:259-263, 1972. B.J. Gurland, N.J. Yorkston, K. Goldberg, J.L. Fliess, R.B. Sloane, and A.H. Cristol. "The structured and scaled interview to assess maladjustment (SSIAM). II. Factor analysis, reliability, and validity." *Archives of General Psychiatry* 27:264-267, 1972.

8. R.A. Harper. *Psychoanalysis and Psychotherapy*. Englewood Cliffs: Prentice-Hall, 1959.

9. A. Janov. *The Primal Scream; Primal Therapy: The Cure for Neurosis*. New York: Putnam, 1970.

10. Redlich and Freedman, *Psychiatry*, p. 280.

11. Wolberg, *Psychotherapy*.

12. S. Rosenzweig. "Some implicit common factors in diverse methods of psychotherapy." *American Journal of Orthopsychiatry* 6:412-415, 1936.

## 2. How Psychotherapy Has Been Studied

1. H. Strupp and A.E. Bergin. "Some empirical and conceptual bases for coordinated research in psychotherapy." *International Journal of Psychiatry* 7:20, 1969.

2. H. Strupp and A.E. Bergin. *Research in Individual Psychotherapy: A Bibliography*. Chevy Chase, Maryland: National Institute of Mental Health, 1972.

3. J. Meltzoff and M. Kornreich. *Research in Psychotherapy*. New York: Atherton, 1970.

4. A.E. Bergin. "The evaluation of therapeutic outcome." In A.E. Bergin and S.L. Garfield. *Handbook of Psychotherapy and Behavior Change*. New York: Wiley, 1971.

5. H.J. Eysenck. "The effects of psychotherapy: An evaluation." *Journal of Consulting Psychology* 16:319-324, 1952.

6. L. Luborsky, A.H. Auerbach, M. Chandler, J. Cohen, H.M. Bachrach. "Factors influencing the outcome of psychotherapy." *Psychological bulletin* 75:145-185, 1971.

7. D.H. Malan. "The outcome problem in psychotherapy research." *Archives of General Psychiatry* 29:719-729, 1973.

8. S. Orgel. "Effects of psychoanalysis on the course of peptic ulcer." *Psychosomatic Medicine* 20:117-125, 1958.

9. O.F. Kernberg, *et al.* "Psychotherapy and psychoanalysis: Final report of the Menninger Foundation's Psychotherapy Research Project. *Bull Menninger Clin* 36:No. 1 and 2, 1972.

10. L. Kessel and H.T. Hyman. "The value of psychoanalysis as a therapeutic procedure." *Journal of American Medical Association* 101:1612-1615, 1933.

11. Quoted by John Ball. Personal communication, March 1972.

12. D.W. Fiske, *et al.* "Planning of research on effectiveness of psychotherapy." *Archives of General Psychiatry* 22:22-32, 1970.

13. P.E. Meehl. "Psychotherapy." *Annual Review of Psychology*. Palo Alto: Annual Reviews, 1955.

14. H.J. Eysenck. "The effects of psychotherapy." In H.J. Eysenck, ed. *Handbook of Abnormal Psychology*. New York, Basic Books, 1961.

15. S.B. Sells. "Problems of criteria and validity in diagnosis and therapy." *Journal of Clinical Psychology* 8:23-28, 1952.

16. Eysenck, "Effects of Psychotherapy."

17. C. Landis. "Statistical evaluation of psychotherapeutic methods." In S.E. Hinsie, ed. *Concepts and Problems of Psychotherapy*. London: Heineman, 1938.

18. P.G. Denker. "Results of treatment of psychoneuroses by the general practitioner. A follow-up of 500 cases." *New York State Journal of Medicine* 46:2164-2166, 1946.

19. Bergin, "Therapeutic Outcome."

20. S. Rachman. *The Effects of Psychotherapy*. Oxford, England, Pergamon Press, 1971.

21. D.W. Goodwin. "Follow-up studies of obsessional neurosis." *Archives of General Psychiatry* 20:182, 1967.

22. P. Errera and J.V. Coleman. "A long-term follow-up study of neurotic phobic patients in a psychiatric clinic." *Journal of Nervous and Mental Disease* 136:267-271, 1963.

23. C.E. Schorer, P. Lowinger, T. Sullivan, G.H. Hartlaub. "Improvement without treatment." *Diseases of the Nervous System* 29:100-104, 1968.

24. F. Barron, and T.F. Leary. "Changes in psychoneurotic patients with and without psychotherapy." *Journal of Consulting Psychology* 19:239-245, 1955.

25. Goodwin. "Obsessional Neurosis."

26. Bergin. "Therapeutic Outcome."

27. H. J. Schlesinger. "Problems of doing research on the therapeutic process in psychoanalysis." *Journal of the American Psychoanalytic Association* 22: 1:3-13, 1974.

28. D. A. Hamburg, G. L. Bibring, C. Fisher, A. H. Stanton, R. S. Wallerstein, H. I. Weinstock, and E. Haggard. "Report of Ad Hoc Committee on Central Fact-Gathering Data of the American Psychoanalytic Association." *Journal of the American Psychoanalytic Association* 15:841-861, 1967.

29. Rachman, *Effects of Psychotherapy*.

30. I. Bieber. *Homosexuality: A Psychoanalytic Study*. New York: Basic Books, 1962.

31. J.T. Barendregt. *Research in Psychodiagnostics*. Paris: Mouton, 1961.

32. H. Klein. "A study of changes occurring in patients during and after psychoanalytic treatment." *Current Approaches to Psychoanalysis*. New York: Grune & Stratton, 1960

33. J.Cremerius. *Die Beurteilung des Behandlungserfolges in der Psychotherapie*. Berlin: Springer Verlag, 1962.

34. H.J. Eysenck. *The Effects of Psychotherapy*. New York: Science House Inc., 1969.

35. Rachman, *Effects of Psychotherapy*.

36. Eysenck, *Effects of Psychotherapy*.

37. J.J. Weber, J. Elinson, and L.M. Moss. "The application of ego strength scales to psychoanalytic clinic records." In G.S. Goldman, and D. Shapiro, eds. *Developments in Psychoanalysis at Columbia University: Proceedings of the Twentieth Anniversary Conference*. New York: Columbia Psychoanalytic Clinic for Training and Research, 1965.

38. R.R. Koegler and N.T. Brill. *Treatment of Psychiatric Outpatients*. New York: Appleton-Century-Crofts, 1967.

39. D. Cappon. "Results of psychotherapy." *British Journal of Psychiatry* 110:35-45, 1964.

40. M. Rosenbaum, J. Friedlander, and S.M. Kaplan. "Evaluation of results of psychotherapy." *Psychosomatic Medicine* 18:113-132, 1956.

41. D.H. Malan. *A Study of Brief Psychotherapy*. Springfield: Thomas, 1963.

42. D.H. Malan. "The outcome problem in psychotherapy research." *Archives of General Psychiatry* 29:719-729, 1973.

43. P. London. *Modes and Morals of Psychotherapy*. New York: Holt, Rinehart & Winston, 1964.

44. H.J. Eysenck and H.R. Beech. "Counter conditioning and related methods." In *Handbook of Psychotherapy and Behavior Change*. A.E. Bergin and S.L. Garfield. New York: Wiley, 1971, p. 600.

45. J. Wolpe, *Psychotherapy by Reciprocal Inhibition*. Stanford: Stanford University Press, 1958.

46. A. Lazarus. "The results of behavior therapy in 126 cases of severe neurosis." *Behavior Research and Therapy* 1:69-79, 1963.

47. T.G. Stampfl and D.J. Levis. "Essentials of implosive therapy: A learning-theory-based psychodynamic behavioral therapy." *Journal of Abnormal Psychology* 72:496-503, 1967.

48. B. Saper. "A report on behavior therapy with outpatient clinic patients." *Psychiatric Quarterly* 45:209-215, 1971.

49. S. Rachman, R. Hodgson, and I.M. Marks. "The treatment of chronic obsessive-compulsive neurosis." *Behavior Research and Therapy* 9:237-247, 1971.

50. A. Hussain. "Behavior therapy in 105 cases." In J. Wolpe, A. Salter, and L.J. Reyna, eds. *The Conditioning Therapies: The Challenge in Psychotherapy*. New York: Holt, 1963, pp. 54-61.

51. G. Paul. *Insight vs. Desensitization in Psychotherapy*. Stanford: Stanford University Press, 1966.

52. A. DiLoreto. *Comparative Psychotherapy*. New York: Aldine-Atherton, 1971.

53. G. Paul. "Insight versus desensitization in psychotherapy two years after termination." *Journal of Consulting Psychology* 31:333-348, 1967.

54. A.R. Stone, *et al.* "An intensive five-year follow-up study of treated psychiatric patients." *Journal of Nervous and Mental Disease* 133:410-422, 1961.

55. E.C. Land. "A comparison of patient improvement resulting from two therapeutic techniques." *Dissertation Abstracts* 25:628, 1964.

56. M. Straker. "Brief psychotherapy in an outpatient clinic:

Evolution and evaluation." *American Journal of Psychiatry* 124:1219-1225, 1968.

57. W. Schofield. "Changes in response to the MMPI following certain therapies." *Psychological Monographs* 64:(Whole No. 311), 1950.

58. W. Schofield. "A further study of the effects of therapies on MMPI responses." *Journal of Abnormal and Social Psychology* 48:67-77, 1953.

59. M.G. Gelder, I.M. Marks, and H.H. Wolff. "Desensitization and psychotherapy in the treatment of phobic states: A controlled inquiry." *British Journal of Psychiatry* 113:53-73, 1967.

60. M.G. Gelder and I.M. Marks. "Severe agoraphobia: A controlled prospective trial of behavior therapy." *British Journal of Psychiatry* 112:309-319, 1966.

61. I.M. Marks and M.G. Gelder. "A controlled retrospective study of behavior therapy in phobic patients." *British Journal of Psychiatry* 111:561-573, 1965.

62. J.E. Cooper, M.G. Gelder, and I.M. Marks. "Results of behavior therapy in seventy-seven psychiatric patients." *British Medical Journal* 1:1222-1225, 1965.

63. J.E. Cooper. "A study of behavior therapy in thirty psychiatric patients." *Lancet* 1:411-415, 1963.

64. A. Bandura, E.B. Blanchard, and B. Ritter. "The relative efficacy of desensitization and modeling approaches for inducing behavioral, affective, and attitudinal changes." *Journal of Personality and Social Psychology* 13:173-199, 1969.

65. H. Leitenberg, W.F. Agras, and L.E. Thomson. "A sequential analysis of the effect of selective positive reinforcement in modifying anorexia nervosa." *Behavior Research and Therapy* 6:211-218, 1968.

66. G.C. Davison. "Systematic desensitization as a counter conditioning process." *Journal of Abnormal Psychology* 73:91-99, 1968.

67. L. Krasner. "The therapist as a social reinforcer; Man or machine." Presented at American Psychological Association, Philadelphia, 1963.

68. A.E. Bergin and L.G. Jasper. "Correlates of empathy in psychotherapy: A replication." *Journal of Abnormal Psychology*

74:477-481, 1969.

69. D.H. Frayn. "A relationship between rated ability and personality traits in psychotherapists." *American Journal of Psychiatry* 124:1232-1237, 1968.

70. R.R. Holt and L. Luborsky. *Personality Patterns of Psychiatrists: A study in Selection Techniques*. New York: Basic Books, 1958.

71. B. Betz and J.C. Whitehorn. "The relationship of the therapist to the outcome of therapy in schizophrenia." *Psychiatric Research Reports* 5:89-105, 1956.

72. A.M. Razin. "A-B variable in psychotherapy: A critical review." *Psychological Bulletin* 75:1-21, 1971.

73. G.M. Chartier. "A-B therapist variable: Real or imagined?" *Psychological Bulletin* 75:22-33, 1971.

74. D.M. McNair, D.M. Callahan, and M. Lorr. "Therapist type and patient response to psychotherapy." *Journal of Consulting Psychology* 26:425-429, 1962.

75. R.D. Cartwright and J.L. Vogel. "A comparison of changes in psychoneurotic patients during matched periods of therapy and no therapy." *Journal of Consulting Psychology* 24:121-127, 1960.

76. M.M. Katz, M. Lorr, and E.A. Rubinstein. "Remainer patient attributes and their relation to subsequent improvement in psychotherapy." *Journal of Consulting Psychology* 23:411-413, 1958.

77. D.W. Boulware. "Preferences and expectancies regarding therapist age and sex." *Dissertation Abstracts* 30:3381-B, 1970.

78. L.C. Hartlage. "Sub-professional therapists' use of reinforcement versus traditional psychotherapeutic techniques with schizophrenics." *Journal of Consulting and Clinical Psychology* 34:181, 1970.

79. V. Patterson, H. Levene, and L. Breger. Treatment and training outcomes with two time-limited therapies. *Archives of General Psychiatry* 25:161, 1971.

80. F.E. Fiedler. "The concept of an ideal therapeutic relationship." *Journal of Consulting Psychology* 14:239-245, 1950.

81. W. Schofield. *Psychotherapy: The Purchase of Friendship*. Englewood Cliffs: Prentice-Hall, 1964.

82. E.B. Gallagher, M.R. Sharaf, and D.J. Levinson. "The influ-

ence of patient and therapist in determining the use of psychotherapy in a hospital setting." *Psychiatry* 28:297-310, 1965.

83. P.L. Lowinger and S. Dobie. "Attitudes and emotions of the psychiatrist in the initial interview." *American Journal of Psychotherapy* 20:17-34, 1966.

84. E.H. Nash *et al.* "Systematic preparation of patients for short-term psychotherapy." *Journal of Nervous and Mental Disease* 140:374-383, 1965.

85. S.D. Imber, E.H. Nash, and A.R. Stone. "Social class and duration of psychotherapy." *Journal of Clinical Psychology* 11:281-284, 1955.

86. M. Lorr, M.M. Katz, and E.A. Rubinstein. "The prediction of length of stay in psychotherapy." *Journal of Consulting Psychology* 22:321-327, 1958.

87. S.T. Michael. "Social class and psychiatric treatment." *Journal of Psychiatric Research* 5:243-254, 1967.

88. J. Yamamoto. "Cultural problems in psychiatric therapy." *Archives of General Psychiatry* 19:45-49, 1968.

89. A.P. Goldstein, K. Heller, and L.B. Sechrest. *Psychotherapy and the Psychology of Behavior Change*. New York: Wiley, 1966.

90. H.J. Cross. "The outcome of psychotherapy: A selected analysis of research findings." *Journal of Consulting Psychology* 28:311-316, 1964.

91. J.I. Novick. *The Effectiveness of Brief Psychotherapy as a Function of Ego Strength*. Doctoral Dissertation, New York University, Ann Arbor: University Microfilms, 1961.

92. R.E. Harris and C. Christiansen. "Prediction of response to brief psychotherapy." *Journal of Psychology* 21:269-284, 1946.

93. P.T. Annesley. "Psychiatric illness in adolescence: Presentation and prognosis." *Journal of Mental Science* 107:268-278, 1961.

94. R. Feldman, M. Lorr, and S.B. Russell. "A mental hygiene clinic case survey." *Journal of Clinical Psychology* 14:245-250, 1958.

95. K.E. Appel *et al.* "Long-term psychotherapy." *Research Publications of the Association for Research in Nervous and Mental Disease* 31:21-34, 1951.

96. M.J. Tissenbaum. "Psychotherapy in a mental hygiene clinic." *Psychiatric Quarterly* 28:465-478, 1954.

97. M.S. Wallach and H.H. Strupp. "Psychotherapists' clinical judgments and attitudes toward patients." *Journal of Consulting Psychology* 24:316-323, 1960.

98. A. Raskin. "Factors therapists associate with motivation to enter psychotherapy." *Journal of Clinical Psychology* 17:62-65, 1961.

99. H.H. Strupp, R.E. Fox, and K. Lessler. *Patients View Their Psychotherapy*. Baltimore: Johns Hopkins University Press, 1969.

100. Malan, *Brief Psychotherapy*.

101. J.D. Frank, *Persuasion and Healing: A Comparative Study of Psychotherapy*. Baltimore: Johns Hopkins University Press, 1961.

102. A.R. Stone *et al.* "Some situational factors associated with response to psychotherapy." *American Journal of Orthopsychiatry* 35:682-687, 1965.

103. P.L. Lowinger and S. Dobie. "Attitudes and emotions of the psychiatrist in the initial interview." *American Journal of Psychotherapy* 20:17-34, 1966.

104. W. Gerler. "Outcome of psychotherapy as a function of client-counselor similarity." *Dissertation Abstracts* 18:1864, 1958.

105. R.C. Carson and R.W. Heine. "Similarity and success in therapeutic dyads." *Journal of Consulting Psychology* 26:38-43, 1962.

106. E. Lichtenstein. "Personality similarity and therapeutic success: A failure to replicate." *Journal of Consulting Psychology* 30:282, 1966.

107. R.C. Carson and C.E. Llewellyn. "Similarity in therapeutic dyads: A re-evaluation." *Journal of Consulting Psychology* 30:458, 1966.

108. C.B. Truax *et al.* "Therapist empathy, genuineness and warmth, and patient outcome." *Journal of Consulting Psychology* 30:395-401, 1966.

109. N. Muehlberg, R. Pierce, and J. Drasgow. "A factor analysis of therapeutically facilitative conditions." *Journal of Clinical Psychology* 25:93-95, 1969.

110. M. Lorr. "Client perceptions of therapists: A study of the therapeutic relation." *Journal of Consulting Psychology* 29:146-149, 1965.

111. F.R. Staples and R.B. Sloane. "Relation of speech patterns in psychotherapy to empathic ability, responsiveness to approval and disapproval." *Diseases of the Nervous System* 31:100-104, 1970.

112. F.R. Staples and R.B. Sloane. "Truax variables, speech patterns, and therapeutic outcome." Unpublished manuscript, 1969.

## 3. The Plan of the Study

1. B.J. Gurland, N.J. Yorkston, A.R. Stone, J.D. Frank, and J. L. Fliess. "The structured and scaled interview to assess maladjustment (SSIAM). I. Description, rationale and development." *Archives of General Psychiatry* 27:259-263, 1972. B.J. Gurland, N.J. Yorkston, K. Goldberg, J.L. Fliess, R.B. Sloane, and A.H. Cristol. "The structured and scaled interview to assess maladjustment (SSIAM). II. Factor analysis, reliability and validity." *Archives of General Psychiatry* 27:264-267, 1972.

2. R.B. Sloane, A.H. Cristol, M.C. Pepernik, and F.R. Staples, "Role preparation and expectation of improvement in psychotherapy." *Journal of Nervous and Mental Disease* 150:18-26, 1970.

## 4. Outcome of Treatment at Four Months

1. B.J. Gurland, N.J. Yorkston, A.R. Stone, J.D. Frank, and J.L. Fliess. "The structured and scaled interview to assess maladjustment (SSIAM). I. Description, rationale, and development." *Archives of General Psychiatry* 27:259-263, 1972.

2. B.J. Gurland, N.J. Yorkston, K. Goldberg, J.L. Fliess, R.B. Sloane, and A.H. Cristol. "The structured and scaled interview to assess maladjustment (SSIAM). II. Factor analysis, reliability, and validity." *Archives of General Psychiatry* 27:264-267, 1972.

3. A.E. Bergin. "The evaluation of therapeutic outcomes." In A.E. Bergin and S.L. Garfield, eds. *Handbook of Psychotherapy and Behavior Change*. New York:Wiley, 1971, p. 241.

5. Follow-Up Evaluations

1. J.D. Frank. *Persuasion and Healing: A Comparative Study of Psychotherapy*. Baltimore: Johns Hopkins University Press, 1961.
2. A.A. Lazarus. *Behavior Therapy and Beyond*. New York: McGraw-Hill, 1972.
3. A.P. Goldstein. *Therapist-Patient Expectancies in Psychotherapy*. New York: Pergamon Press, 1962.

6. Differences Between Behavior Therapy and Psychotherapy

1. C.B. Truax and R.R. Carkhuff. *Toward Effective Counseling and Psychotherapy: Training and Practice*. Chicago: Aldine, 1967.
2. H.L. Lennard and A. Bernstein. *The Anatomy of Psychotherapy*. New York: Columbia University Press, 1960.
3. J.D. Matarazzo. "The interview." In B.J. Wolman, ed. *Handbook of Clinical Psychology*. New York: McGraw-Hill, 1965.
4. D.H. Malan. "The outcome problem in psychotherapy research." *Archives of General Psychiatry* 29: 719-729, 1973.
5. M. Lorr. "Client perceptions of therapists: A study of the therapeutic relation." *Journal of Consulting Psychology* 29:146-149, 1965.
6. F.E. Fiedler. "The concept of an ideal therapeutic relationship," *Journal of Consulting Psychology* 14:239-245, 1950.

7. Patient Characteristics, Process Measures, and Outcome

1. H. H. Strupp and A. Bergin. "Some empirical and conceptual bases for coordinated research in psychotherapy." *International Journal of Psychiatry* 7:18-90, 1969.
2. J. Meltzoff and M. Kornreich. *Research in Psychotherapy*. New York: Atherton, 1970, pp. 204-264.
3. L. Luborsky, M. Chandler, A.H. Auerbach, J. Cohen, and H. M. Bachrach. "Factors influencing the outcome of psychotherapy: a review of quantitative research." *Psychological Bulletin* 75: 145-185, 1971.

4. C.B. Truax and R.R. Carkhuff. *Toward Effective Counseling and Psychotherapy: Training and Practice*. Chicago: Aldine, 1967.

5. Richard A. Prager and S.L. Garfield. "Client initial disturbance and outcome in psychotherapy." In I.M. Marks, E. Bergin, *et al. Psychotherapy and Behavior Change*. Chicago: Aldine, 1972, pp. 70-75.

6. A.O. DiLoreto. *Comparative Psychotherapy*. Chicago: Aldine-Atherton, 1971.

7. C.B. Truax, D.G. Wargo, J.D. Frank, S.D. Imber, C.C. Battle, R. Hoehn-Saric, E. Nash, and A. Stone. "Therapist empathy, genuineness, and warmth and patient therapeutic outcome." *Journal of Consulting Psychology* 30:395-401, 1966.

8. S.L. Garfield and A.E. Bergin. "Therapeutic conditions and outcome." *Journal of Abnormal Psychology* 77:108-114, 1971.

9. C.B. Truax *et al.* "Therapist Empathy."

10. C.B. Truax and K.M. Mitchell. "Research on certain therapists interpersonal skills in relation to process and outcome." In A.E. Bergin and S.L. Garfield. *Handbook of Psychotherapy and Behavior Change*. New York: Wiley, 1971, pp. 299-344.

11. D.H. Malan. "The outcome problem in psychotherapy research." *Archives of General Psychiatry* 29:719-729, 1973.

12. I.M. Marks and M.G. Gelder. "Common ground between behavior therapy and psychodynamic methods." *British Journal of Medical Psychology* 39:11-23, 1966.

13. V.L. Ryan and M.N. Gizynski. "Behavior therapy in retrospect." *Journal of Consulting and Clinical Psychology* 37:1-9, 1971.

14. W. Schofield. *Psychotherapy; The Purchase of Friendship*. Englewood Cliffs: Prentice-Hall, 1964, p. 133.

15. Luborsky *et al.* "Outcome of psychotherapy," p. 149.

16. Meltzoff and Kornreich, *Research in Psychotherapy*, p. 208-211.

17. D.C. Conrad. "An empirical study of the concept of psychotherapeutic success." *Journal of Consulting Psychology* 16:92-97, 1952.

18. L.A. Gottschalk, P. Mayerson, and A. Gottleib. "Prediction and evaluation of outcome in an emergency brief psychotherapy clinic." *Journal of Nervous and Mental Disease* 144:77-96, 1967.

19. E. Uhlenhuth and D. Duncan. "Subjective change in psychoneurotic outpatients with medical student therapists. II. Some determinants of change." *Archives of General Psychiatry* 18:532-540, 1968.

20. Strupp and Bergin, "Coordinated research," p. 87.

21. F.R. Staples and R.B. Sloane. "Truax variables, speech patterns, and therapeutic outcome." Unpublished manuscript, 1969.

# INDEX

A-B therapist variable, 41-42, 80
Accurate empathy. *See* Relationship Questionnaire; Truax variables
Adjustment measures. *See* Structured and Scaled Interview to Assess Maladjustment
American Psychoanalytic Association, study of psychoanalytic effectiveness, 23-24
Anxiety, 97-99, 210
Assessors, 51-52
Assignment to treatment groups, 73-76, 235-236
Behavior therapy: definition of, 9-12, 81-82, 237-240; studies of effectiveness of, 27-28
Bergin, A. E., 15, 16-17, 21
Case histories, 58, 76-79, 112-115, 131-135
Chartier, G. M., 41-42
Clinical techniques: comparison of, 168-169; patients' ratings of importance of, 206-208
Content of therapy interview. *See* Temple Content Categories
Control group. *See* Wait list
Countertransference. *See* Therapist Attitude toward Patient
Depth of interpersonal contact. *See* Truax variables
DiLoreto, A. O., 34-38
Directiveness. *See* Lennard and Bernstein Categories; Lorr Scale; Temple Content Categories
Egodystonia, 210

Emotional disturbance, 210
Expectations of treatment, 204
Extraversion, 183-185
Eysenck, H. J., 16, 20-21
Figures, explanation of, 147, 175
Gelder, M. G., 39-40
Graphs, explanation of, 147, 175
Improvement measures. *See* Outcome measures
Interaction, patient-therapist, 170-172, *See also* Lennard and Bernstein Categories; Lorr Scale; Patient Questionnaire; Relationship Questionnaire; Speech patterns; Temple Content Categories; Therapist Attitude toward Patient; Truax variables
Inter-rater comparisons, 107-112
Kornreich, M., 15
Lennard and Berstein Categories: samples rated, 146; description of, 150-151; and symptomatic improvement, 194-196; definition of, 243-244
Lorr Scale, 163-166, 202
Luborsky, L., 17
Malan, D. H., 17, 26-27
Marks, I. M., 39-40
Measures of improvement. *See* Outcome measures
Meltzoff, J., 15
Minimal contact group. *See* Wait list
Neuroticism, 93-94
Nonlexical speech characteristics. *See* Speech patterns
Outcome measures, 52-54, 70-72, 85-86, 174
Overall improvement: assessors' ratings of, 100-103; patients' ratings at four months, 103-106; patients' ratings at one year, 136-137
Patient characteristics: in literature, 43-45; MMPI, 176-178; severity of initial disturbance, 178-182; personality characteristics, 182-185; type of target symptom, 186-188; demographic characteristics, 188-190
Patient perception of therapist. *See* Lorr Scale; Patient Questionnaire; Relationship Questionnaire
Patients, anecdotal accounts of, 58, 76-79, 112-115, 131-135

Patient Questionnaire, 202-208
Patient sample, 54-64, 70
Patient-therapist interaction. *See* Interaction, patient-therapist
Paul, G. L., 29-34
Process variables, 82, 170-172, *See also* Lennard and Bernstein Categories; Lorr Scale; Patient Questionnaire; Relationship Questionnaire; Speech patterns; Temple Content Categories; Therapist Attitude toward Patient; Truax variables
Psychoanalytically oriented psychotherapy: definition of, 8-9, 81-82, 237-240; studies of effectiveness of, 22-27
Psychotherapy. *See* Psychoanalytically oriented psychotherapy
Rachman, S., 24-25
Razin, A. M., 41
Redlich, F. C., 8-9
Relationship, patient-therapist. *See* Interaction, patient-therapist
Relationship Questionnaire (Truax and Carkhuff), 162-163, 200-202
Self-congruence, *See* Truax variables
Sex, effects of, 93-94, 97
Speech patterns, 46-47, 152-156, 193-194
Spontaneous improvement of outpatients, 20-22, 103
Strategies, therapeutic. *See* Clinical techniques
Structured and Scaled Interview to Assess Maladjustment (SSIAM): description of, 5-6, 54, 90-92, 299-233; improvement at four months, 92; comparisons between groups' improvement, 93-94; effects of sex and neuroticism on improvement, 93-94; effect of therapist experience on improvement, 95; improvement at one year, 119-121; improvement of "terminators" at one year, 131; improvement at two years, 135-136
Strupp, H., 15
Symptom substitution, 5, 28, 100
Systematic desensitization, 9-10
Target symptom: 52-54, 64-70
Target symptom improvement, 87-90, 93-94, 95; at four months, 87; at one year, 119-121; of "terminators," 129; at two years, 135-136
Temple Content Categories, 157-160, 196-198
"Terminators" versus "continuers," 121-129

Therapist Attitude toward Patient, 160-162, 198-200
Therapist experience, 42-43, 95, 166-167
Therapists, 79-80
Therapist variables, 41-43, 80
Time limitation, 204-206
"Transference-parent link," 27, 197-198
Truax variables, 146-149, 190-192, *See also* Lorr Scale; Relationship Questionnaire
Unconditional positive regard. *See* Truax variables
Wait list, 83-84
YAVIS syndrome, 43, 190, 209

Bei Fragen zur Produktsicherheit wenden Sie sich bitte an:
If you have any questions regarding product safety,
please contact:

Walter de Gruyter GmbH
Genthiner Straße 13
10785 Berlin
productsafety@degruyterbrill.com